THE
EVERYTHING®
VEGAN PREGNANCY BOOK

Dear Reader,

When I had my two daughters, there were no books on vegan pregnancy. Even though I knew that I was eating well, I wished there was something I could turn to for advice. Perhaps because of those experiences, life-cycle vegan/vegetarian nutrition has been the area I've specialized in. I've gotten late-night phone calls from pregnant vegans and have been approached by other dietitians with questions about vegan pregnancy. As a long-term vegan, I'm happy to support others who are interested in this path. I hope that you'll learn from this book and turn to it when you have questions.

Your pregnancy is yours to shape. If you're a first-time mom, you'll be getting lots of experience with decision making when there isn't a clear right or wrong answer. That's good practice for raising children. Gather information, talk to people you trust, and then make the best decisions you can.

This time goes so quickly. Keep a journal, take pictures, try to live in the moment and know that you're making a difference, both by having a child and by being vegan.

Best wishes to you and your family,

Reed Mangels

Welcome to the EVERYTHING® Series!

These handy, accessible books give you all you need to tackle a difficult project, gain a new hobby, comprehend a fascinating topic, prepare for an exam, or even brush up on something you learned back in school but have since forgotten.

You can choose to read an Everything® book from cover to cover or just pick out the information you want from our four useful boxes: e-questions, e-facts, e-alerts, and e-ssentials.

We give you everything you need to know on the subject, but throw in a lot of fun stuff along the way, too.

We now have more than 400 Everything® books in print, spanning such wide-ranging categories as weddings, pregnancy, cooking, music instruction, foreign language, crafts, pets, New Age, and so much more. When you're done reading them all, you can finally say you know Everything®!

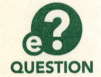

QUESTION

Answers to common questions

FACT

Important snippets of information

ALERT

Urgent warnings

ESSENTIAL

Quick handy tips

PUBLISHER Karen Cooper

DIRECTOR OF ACQUISITIONS AND INNOVATION Paula Munier

MANAGING EDITOR, EVERYTHING® SERIES Lisa Laing

COPY CHIEF Casey Ebert

ASSISTANT PRODUCTION EDITOR Jacob Erickson

ACQUISITIONS EDITOR Brett Palana-Shanahan

SENIOR DEVELOPMENT EDITOR Brett Palana-Shanahan

EDITORIAL ASSISTANT Ross Weisman

EVERYTHING® SERIES COVER DESIGNER Erin Alexander

LAYOUT DESIGNERS Colleen Cunningham, Elisabeth Lariviere, Ashley Vierra, Denise Wallace

Visit the entire Everything® series at www.everything.com

THE
EVERYTHING®
VEGAN PREGNANCY BOOK

All you need to know for a healthy
pregnancy that fits your lifestyle

Reed Mangels, PhD, RD, LD, FADA

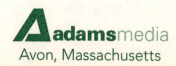

Avon, Massachusetts

For Arnie, Sarah, and Leah, with love.

An Everything® Series Book.
Everything® and everything.com® are registered trademarks of F+W Media, Inc.

Published by Adams Media, a division of F+W Media, Inc.
57 Littlefield Street, Avon, MA 02322 U.S.A.
www.adamsmedia.com

The Everything® Vegan Pregnancy Book contains material adapted and abridged from:
The Everything® Pregnancy Book, 3rd Edition by Paula Ford-Martin, copyright © 2007 by F+W Media, Inc.,
ISBN 10: 1-59869-286-0; ISBN 13: 978-1-59869-286-0; and *The Everything® Vegan Cookbook,* by Jolinda
Hackett with Lorena Novak Bull, RD, copyright © 2010 by F+W Media, Inc., ISBN 10: 1-4405-0216-1;
ISBN 13: 978-1-4405-0216-3

ISBN 10: 1-4405-2551-X
ISBN 13: 978-1-4405-2551-3
eISBN 10: 1-4405-2607-9
eISBN 13: 978-1-4405-2607-7

Printed in the United States of America.

10 9 8 7 6 5 4 3 2 1

Library of Congress Cataloging-in-Publication Data
is available from the publisher.

The Everything® Vegan Pregnancy Book does not purport to render medical advice. Every pregnant woman should consult her professional health-care provider for such advice.

This publication is designed to provide accurate and authoritative information with regard to the subject matter covered. It is sold with the understanding that the publisher is not engaged in rendering legal, accounting, or other professional advice. If legal advice or other expert assistance is required, the services of a competent professional person should be sought.
—From a *Declaration of Principles* jointly adopted by a Committee of the American Bar Association and a Committee of Publishers and Associations

Many of the designations used by manufacturers and sellers to distinguish their products are claimed as trademarks. Where those designations appear in this book and Adams Media was aware of a trademark claim, the designations have been printed with initial capital letters.

This book is available at quantity discounts for bulk purchases.
For information, please call 1-800-289-0963.

Contents

Acknowledgments

Thank you to Brett Palana-Shanahan, editor, for always answering my questions. Thanks also to Paula Ford-Martin, author of *The Everything*® *Pregnancy Book*, and Jolinda Hackett, author of *The Everything*® *Vegan Cookbook*, for the use of some of the materials they developed. Much appreciation to Charles Stahler and Debra Wasserman of The Vegetarian Resource Group for their inspiration, and to Ginny Messina, MPH, RD and Winston Craig, PhD, RD for many years of productive discussions about vegan nutrition. Finally, thanks to my husband, daughters, brothers, and parents for their ongoing support and encouragement.

Top 10 Things You Need to Know
for a Healthy Vegan Pregnancy

1. A well-planned vegan diet can meet your baby's nutritional needs as well as your own.

2. Eating a variety of healthy vegan foods keeps things interesting and makes it more likely that you're getting the nutrients you need.

3. Use a reliable source of vitamin B_{12} (fortified food and/or supplement) every day.

4. People are likely to ask you questions about your diet; try not to stress about it. Your food choices are kind to animals and the earth.

5. Prenatal supplements are good insurance.

6. Be sure you know where you get your protein—you'll be asked about this often.

7. A healthy amount of weight gain (assuming your weight was normal before you were pregnant) is 25–35 pounds.

8. Iron deficiency occurs frequently in pregnancy and is not unique to vegans. Choose high-iron foods and take an iron supplement if your provider recommends it.

9. Alcohol and tobacco should be avoided during pregnancy.

10. Whole grains, dried beans, fruits, vegetables, and nuts and seeds are the foundation of a healthy vegan diet.

Introduction

IT'S A GREAT TIME to be vegan. Many supermarkets carry specialty vegan foods that were once difficult to find. You can choose between vegan samosas, chorizo, hot and sour soup, and all sorts of other prepared and convenience foods. Gone are the days of steamed vegetable plates—restaurants, bakeries, cafeterias, and other eating establishments feature creative vegan dishes. Vegan cookbooks and blogs abound.

Attitudes toward vegan diets have changed as well. People used to say, "Vegan diets are all right for adults but not for pregnant women or children." These days, more and more women are realizing that a vegan diet is a healthy way to eat during pregnancy and that there's no reason to stop being vegan just because you're pregnant. Still, you may be feeling a little jittery. You may wonder where you can go to find answers to questions like, "Am I getting enough protein?" and "How am I going to talk to my doctor about being vegan?" Besides questions that are unique to vegans, you also have typical questions that every pregnant woman asks, such as, "Am I doing this right?" "Will I be a good mother?" "Is it safe to wear a seat belt?"

If you're like most vegan women, you don't have a lot of role models—it's not too likely that your mom was vegan when she was pregnant (although it is possible—some families have been lifelong vegans for three or more generations). Vegans are still a small percentage of the population (1 percent to 2 percent of adults, according to the latest polls), so your friends may not have a lot of experience with this either. Although over 4 million American women had babies in 2008, most of them weren't vegan.

This book was designed to answer questions your doctor may not be able to help you with. Keep in mind that the average physician had less than twenty-four hours of nutrition education in four years of medical school, and little or none of this focused on vegan diets. Of course, your health care provider is the best person to talk to about specific medical questions related to your pregnancy.

This book encourages you to talk with your health care provider. You're working together with the goal of a healthy, safe pregnancy and birth. Good communication is key to achieving this goal. Your provider brings experience and medical training to the table; you bring your unique knowledge of your body and your history. You are responsible for educating yourself, asking questions, and making sure you're satisfied with the answers. Remember, you're advocating both for yourself and for your child. The skills that you develop now will be useful as you speak up for your child, from the first visit to the pediatrician to deciding which preschool is best to choosing a college.

This book will meet your needs throughout your pregnancy with a focus on practical how-to information. The science is there, but you won't need an advanced degree to find out what you need to do. You'll learn about vegan nutrition and foods as well as take a tour of the nine months of pregnancy and what happens once baby arrives. The recipes will give you lots of ideas and opportunities to try new foods and vegan versions of some favorite dishes. You can use this book throughout your pregnancy and even afterward to answer questions about vegan nutrition and foods.

CHAPTER 1

Vegan Diets: The Basics

Whether you've been vegan for many years, are a relative newcomer to veganism, or are simply contemplating being vegan, adding pregnancy to the equation may raise questions. Rest assured, the American Dietetic Association (ADA) has said that well-planned vegan diets are "appropriate for all stages of the life cycle including pregnancy and lactation." Pregnancy (or prepregnancy) is a great time to learn more about vegan nutrition so that you can be sure you are making the best possible food choices.

Vegan Defined

The Vegan Society, formed in 1944 and based in the United Kingdom, defines veganism as, "a way of living that seeks to exclude, as far as possible and practicable, all forms of exploitation of, and cruelty to, animals for food, clothing, and any other purpose." The Vegetarian Resource Group, a nonprofit educational group in the United States, says, "Vegetarians do not eat meat, fish, or poultry. Vegans, in addition to being vegetarian, do not use other animal products and by-products such as eggs, dairy products, honey, leather, fur, silk, wool, cosmetics, and soaps derived from animal products."

The sense of both of these definitions is that vegans avoid using animal products or foods or ingredients derived from animal products. Some ingredients derived from animal products may be fairly obvious, such as chicken or beef broth or casein from milk. Other ingredients may be less apparent. Gelatin, for example, is derived from animal bones and connective tissue. Carmine (sometimes called cochineal) is a red food coloring derived from the dried bodies of female beetles. These are examples of ingredients that vegans avoid. Vegans are used to reading ingredient listings on products and making decisions about which products or ingredients fit into their values scheme.

QUESTION

What does it mean when a product is labeled vegan?
There are no federal rules regulating the use of "vegan" on labels. Some private companies and nonprofit organizations have developed their own standards and guidelines as to what a vegan food is. To determine if a food meets your definition of vegan, check the ingredient listing.

Vegans also try to avoid foods that may have used animal products in their production. For example, some sugar companies process sugar through a bone char in order to remove color from the sugar. Wine production may also involve animal products. Clarifying agents for wine include egg whites, casein (from milk), gelatin, and isinglass (from fish). Foods fortified with vitamin D contain one of two forms of vitamin D, D_2, or D_3. Vitamin D_3 is typically made from lanolin, an oily substance from sheep's wool.

What Are Vegan Foods?

Vegans eat a wide variety of foods, many of which are familiar to those eating a more traditional American diet. For example, a vegan breakfast could include orange juice, toast with jelly, oatmeal with raisins, and coffee or tea. Lunch could be a standard PB and J sandwich with an apple and some chips, while dinner could be bean burritos, a tossed salad with Italian dressing, and apple crisp.

Vegans may also choose some foods that can seem less familiar. For instance, breakfast could include vegan "sausage" and pancakes, lunch could feature a veggie burger or dog, and dinner could be barbecued seitan over quinoa with vegan biscuits and a frozen dessert based on coconut milk.

Many foods traditionally made with animal products are available in vegan form in large supermarkets or natural foods stores. From macaroni and cheese to fish sticks to barbecue ribs, there are convenient vegan options.

Vegan cookbooks and websites offer recipes for making your favorite foods vegan. Recipes can include simple tricks like replacing eggs with flaxseed or tofu or feature more complicated formulas to make dishes that taste like seafood or dairy-based cheese.

Many restaurants have vegan options on their menus. If you don't see something that you like, don't hesitate to ask. Chefs are often happy to create a dish that meets your dietary needs. Ethnic restaurants frequently have vegan dishes or dishes that could easily be made vegan. Here are a few ideas:

- Veggie no-cheese pizza—make sure to get lots of your favorite vegetable toppings. Ask if the dough contains cheese, milk, or eggs
- Moo Shu vegetables—ask your server to tell the kitchen to leave out eggs
- Falafel—crunchy chickpea balls in a pita pocket with a spicy sauce
- Indian curries and dahl—ask to be made with oil instead of ghee (clarified butter)
- Bean burritos and tacos—hold the cheese and sour cream; check for lard in refried beans

- Pasta with mushroom or marinara sauce (hold the Parmesan)
- Ethiopian injera and lentil stew

Fitting a Vegan Diet to Your Lifestyle

When you decide to become vegan, there are no specific requirements as to how much (or how little) cooking you will need to do. Some vegans love to prepare meals and create new recipes. They may have shelves of cookbooks and the latest equipment. Other vegans rely on takeout, convenience foods, and quick-to-fix meals. You may find yourself at one of these extremes or somewhere in the middle. You may even vary your style from day to day. You can make a vegan diet fit your food and cooking preferences. If you want to be a foodie, there are plenty of opportunities to try new ingredients and seek out new techniques. If you need to make dinner in twenty minutes, convenience foods like canned beans, precut vegetables, and quick-cooking pasta are just what you need.

FACT

According to a 2009 poll commissioned in the United States by The Vegetarian Resource Group, approximately 1 percent of the adult population consistently follows a vegan diet. Another 1 percent are vegan except for eating honey. That means more than 2 million adults in the United States are vegan. About half of the vegans in the United States are female and half are male.

Key Nutrients

The key to a nutritionally sound vegan diet is actually quite simple. Eating a variety of foods including fruits, vegetables, plenty of leafy greens, whole-grain products, beans, nuts, and seeds virtually ensures that you'll meet most of your nutrient needs. Subsequent chapters will provide additional details about specific nutrients that are important to be aware of.

One nutrient that vegans are often asked about is protein. Although many foods provide some protein, the dried bean family is an especially good way to get protein. From vegetarian baked beans to chili (*sin carne—without meat*) to lentil soup, it's easy to add beans to your diet. Soy products such as tofu, tempeh, soymilk, textured vegetable protein (TVP), and edamame are also high in protein. Don't forget other foods including whole grains, nuts, nut butters, vegetables, potatoes, and seeds (pumpkin, sesame, sunflower, etc.) that are also great ways to add to your protein totals.

Iron and zinc needs are increased in a vegan diet because they are not absorbed as easily from beans and grains. There are some tricks to increase your absorption of these minerals. Including a food with vitamin C (citrus, tomatoes, cabbage, or broccoli, for instance) at most meals can markedly boost iron and zinc absorption. Good sources of iron and zinc for vegans include enriched breakfast cereals, wheat germ, soy products, dried beans, pumpkin and sunflower seeds, and dark chocolate.

FACT

On a per-calorie basis, many of the top iron sources are vegan. For instance, a 100-calorie portion of cooked spinach supplies almost 16 milligrams of iron and 100 calories of Swiss chard provides over 11 milligrams. Compare that to 100 calories of broiled sirloin steak supplying less than a milligram of iron or 100 calories of skim milk with one-tenth of a milligram of iron.

Calcium and vitamin D are important for strong bones. Contrary to what you may have been told, you don't need to have a cow-milk mustache in order to get enough of these nutrients. Some vegan foods are fortified with calcium and vitamin D. Check labels of soymilk and other plant milks to make sure they have vitamin D and calcium added to them. Calcium is also found in foods like dark leafy greens, tofu set with calcium salts, and dried figs. Vitamin D can also be produced by your skin when you're out in the sun. Vegan vitamin D supplements are another way to meet your vitamin D needs. And, of course, exercise is a key requirement for building strong bones.

Vitamin B_{12} cannot be reliably obtained from unfortified vegan foods, but there are vegan foods that are fortified with this important vitamin. Fortified foods include some brands of breakfast cereals, nutritional yeast, plant-based milks, and mock meats. If you're not sure whether or not you're getting enough vitamin B_{12} from fortified foods, a vitamin B_{12} supplement is a wise idea.

Fish and fish oils are often promoted as sources of omega-3 fatty acids. Vegans have other options. You can get omega-3s from flaxseeds, flax oil, walnuts, hemp seeds, and other foods. There are even vegan versions of the omega-3 fatty acids found in fish oil—DHA and EPA.

By making smart food choices, it's easy to eat a healthy vegan diet—one that's good for you, for your baby-to-be, and for the planet.

Reasons for Being Vegan

People choose to be vegan for many different reasons. Some people initially become vegan for health reasons—perhaps they've had a health crisis or want to reduce the risk of their family history of heart disease or cancer. Other people choose not to use any animal products because they know that there are alternatives that do not involve hurting animals. People's reasons for being vegan may evolve over time also. For example, someone who originally became vegan due to concerns about animals notices significant health benefits from a vegan diet. Someone who became vegan following a heart attack may go on to read more about factory farms and continue to be vegan to help animals as well.

Every year, over 9 million chickens and turkeys are slaughtered in the United States. More than 100 million cattle, pigs, and sheep are killed annually.

For the Animals

Some people choose to be vegan because they believe that eating eggs and dairy products promotes the meat industry. Male chickens not needed for egg production are killed. Male calves are often raised for veal production. And when cows or egg-laying chickens are no longer productive, they are often sold for meat.

Add to these issues the conditions in which many animals are housed, and it is easy to see why people choose not to eat animals or animal by-products. Practices like debeaking, dehorning, castration, and tail docking are routinely carried out. Animals are confined in crowded conditions and are often given hormones to increase production and growth rate. Fishing leads to the death of sea animals that are unintentionally caught and then discarded.

For the Earth

In 2006, the United Nations released an important report assessing livestock's effect on the environment. Livestock production was shown to have a serious effect on land degradation, climate change, air pollution, water shortage and pollution, and the loss of biodiversity. The report concluded that the livestock sector is responsible for a greater production of greenhouse gas than automobiles and other forms of transportation. Livestock also produce almost two-thirds of ammonia emissions, a significant contributor to acid rain.

According to Livestock's Long Shadow, a report by the United Nations, in the United States, livestock are responsible for 55 percent of erosion and sediment, 37 percent of pesticide use, and 50 percent of antibiotic use.

In 2008, Yvo de Boer, head of the United Nations Framework Convention on Climate Change (UNFCCC), summed up a way to solve the environmental problems related to livestock quickly. He said, "The best solution would be for us all to become vegetarians."

For Personal Health

Besides planetary health and health for animals, many vegans recognize significant health benefits from their dietary choices. Vegan diets do not contain cholesterol and are typically low in saturated fats, making them heart-healthy diets. Vegans frequently eat generous amounts of fiber-containing foods like beans, whole grains, and fruits and vegetables. As a group, vegans tend to be leaner than nonvegetarians or nonvegan vegetarians. Vegan diets have been used to treat medical conditions including heart disease and type 2 diabetes.

Other Reasons

While ethics, the environment, and health are the most commonly cited reasons for choosing to be vegan, other motives are also identified. Some people choose to be vegan for reasons related to world hunger. Some become vegan because their loved ones are vegan. Some find a vegan diet to be very economical and choose it as a money-saving technique. Some people want to avoid the hormones and other additives that are frequently introduced into animal products. Some look at veganism as a part of an overall lifestyle committed to nonviolence.

QUESTION

Who are some famous vegetarians?
Famous vegetarians include Leonardo da Vinci, Leo Tolstoy, Albert Einstein, Pythagoras, and Clara Barton. More recently, Janet Jackson, Natalie Portman, Ellen DeGeneres, Moby, Alicia Silverstone, Chelsea Clinton, and Paul McCartney have all embraced vegetarianism. Former President Bill Clinton has tried a mainly vegan diet for heart health and his daughter's wedding featured a vegan wedding cake.

Whatever your reason is for becoming vegan, it's important not to judge other people. How people choose to follow a vegan diet can vary according to their personal beliefs, background, reasons for being vegan, and knowledge level. Be aware that no one is perfect, try to do your best, and avoid being judgemental of others. That's how you can use your lifestyle to promote a more humane and caring world.

Health Benefits

According to the American Dietetic Association's 2009 position paper on vegetarian diets, "appropriately planned vegetarian diets, including total vegetarian or vegan diets, are healthful, nutritionally adequate, and may provide health benefits in the prevention and treatment of certain diseases." There are significant health advantages associated with both vegan and other types of vegetarian diets.

For example, a study in the UK found that both lifelong vegetarians and vegans had lower levels of total and LDL cholesterol in their blood. LDL cholesterol is often referred to as "bad" cholesterol because it is associated with a higher risk of heart disease. When compared to vegetarians who ate eggs and dairy products, vegans had the lowest levels of total and LDL cholesterol. Based on their blood cholesterol levels, the incidence of heart disease might be 24 percent lower in lifelong vegetarians and 57 percent lower in lifelong vegans compared to meat eaters.

High blood pressure also increases the risk of developing heart disease and of having a stroke. Vegans tend to have lower blood pressure than meat eaters and a lower risk of developing hypertension (high blood pressure).

Several studies have used vegan or near-vegan diets to treat people with heart disease. Results have been very positive in terms of modifying risk factors like obesity and LDL cholesterol levels.

FACT

One significant health advantage for vegans is that they tend to have lower body weights than either other vegetarians or meat eaters. Since being overweight increases the risk of developing many chronic diseases including heart disease, type 2 diabetes, high blood pressure, and even breast cancer, the lower average weight seen in vegans is a definite plus.

Vegetarians tend to have a lower overall risk of developing cancers than meat eaters. Research on vegans is limited. One study found that vegans had lower death rates from colorectal cancer, breast cancer, and prostate cancer than did other vegetarians.

Vegans also have lower rates of type 2 diabetes. Type 2 diabetes is the most common form of diabetes. Risk factors for type 2 diabetes include a poor diet, excess weight, and little exercise. Low-fat vegan diets have been successfully used to treat type 2 diabetes.

CHAPTER 2

Getting Ready for Your Vegan Pregnancy

Pregnancy is a time of big changes for you and your family. It's exciting to think about having a new family member. There's a lot to learn as you prepare for parenthood; be patient with yourself. Even before you're pregnant, you can take some positive steps to assure that you're as healthy as possible. Eating well, exercising regularly, and evaluating your lifestyle practices and physical and emotional health are ways to get ready. You can also identify a health care provider you trust who will support you.

Optimizing Weight

If you are planning to have a baby, the American Congress of Obstetricians and Gynecologists (ACOG) recommends you try to reach a healthy weight before becoming pregnant. If you are slightly underweight, gaining a few pounds can help increase the odds that you will become pregnant as well as reducing the risk of having a baby that is too small and that has problems after birth. If you are overweight, reducing weight before becoming pregnant can help reduce your risk of gestational diabetes, high blood pressure, preeclampsia, and caesarean section. Babies whose moms are overweight are at higher risk for developing macrosomia, or a body size of 8 pounds, 13 ounces (4,000 grams) or more, which could make it difficult to pass through the birth canal. Macrosomia also increases the risk of childhood obesity. Since weight loss is not usually recommended during pregnancy, it makes sense to drop a few pounds before becoming pregnant.

If You Need to Gain Weight

As a group, vegans tend to weigh less than nonvegetarians. That's not to say that vegans don't come in every body shape and size possible, but simply that it's more likely you'll weigh somewhat less if you're following a vegan diet. Refer to the table below to see if your prepregnancy weight is considered underweight. If it is, try to gain a few pounds before you become pregnant.

If your height is	If your prepregnant weight is less than this, you are considered underweight
4'10"	91 pounds
4'11"	94 pounds
5'0"	97 pounds
5'1"	100 pounds
5'2"	104 pounds
5'3"	107 pounds
5'4"	110 pounds
5'5"	114 pounds
5'6"	118 pounds
5'7"	121 pounds
5'8"	125 pounds
5'9"	128 pounds

If your height is	If your prepregnant weight is less than this, you are considered underweight
5'10"	132 pounds
5'11"	136 pounds
6'0"	140 pounds

The following ideas are ways to add more calories to your diet, and more calories = weight gain.

- **Be sure you're eating often.** Often means breakfast, lunch, dinner, and one or more substantial snacks. A snack can be as simple as a piece of fruit and a handful of nuts and breakfast can be a bowl of whole-grain cereal with fruit and soymilk.
- **Make beverages count.** Drink smoothies, shakes, fruit or vegetable juices, and hot chocolate (made with fortified soymilk). Water, coffee, and tea are wonderful calorie-free beverages, but when you're trying to gain weight, drink some other beverages also.
- **Indulge a bit.** Sure, you want to eat a healthy diet, but when you're trying to gain a bit of weight, treat yourself to some higher calorie foods—a scoop of nondairy frozen dessert, a vegan cookie or muffin, a granola bar, a handful of trail mix, for instance.
- **Save the salad for last.** Have you ever noticed that when you eat a large salad, suddenly you're not that hungry anymore? It's a great strategy for weight loss, but if you're trying to gain weight, don't fill up on bulky low-calorie foods before you've had a chance to eat other higher calorie foods.
- **Add some oils, nuts, and other high-fat foods.** Ounce for ounce, foods made up mostly of fat are higher calorie foods than starches or protein. Take advantage of this fact and sauté vegetables in olive oil, spread vegan margarine or peanut butter on your breakfast bagel, and add a creamy vegan dressing to your salad.

And, if you're trying to gain a bit of weight before becoming pregnant, take a look at your exercise habits. Exercise is great (more about this soon), but it's probably not the time to spend several hours each day exercising, since you'll need to eat even more to compensate for the calories you expend when you exercise.

If You Need to Lose Weight

Although many vegans are of average weight, there are definitely vegans whose weight is higher than that recommended. If you're in that category, spending a few months focusing on diet and exercise can provide significant benefits in terms of your upcoming pregnancy. Of course, if you're already pregnant, it's not the time to go on a weight-reduction diet.

If your height is	If your prepregnant weight is more than this, you are considered overweight
4'10"	119 pounds
4'11"	124 pounds
5'0"	128 pounds
5'1"	132 pounds
5'2"	136 pounds
5'3"	141 pounds
5'4"	145 pounds
5'5"	150 pounds
5'6"	155 pounds
5'7"	159 pounds
5'8"	164 pounds
5'9"	169 pounds
5'10"	174 pounds
5'11"	179 pounds
6'0"	184 pounds

To reach a healthy weight before pregnancy, focus on healthy foods. Eat plenty of fruits, vegetables, and whole grains every day along with moderate amounts of dried beans and soy products. Limit high-calorie, low-nutrient foods like sweets, sodas, oils, margarine, snack foods, and salad dressings. Remember, improvements that you make with your eating habits now will make it even easier to have a good diet during pregnancy.

You may find it helpful to discuss a weight-reduction diet with a Registered Dietitian (RD), a food and nutrition expert who has met specific academic and professional requirements to qualify for the credential RD.

In addition to the RD credential, your nutrition advisor may have other credentials. Many states have regulatory laws for dietitians and nutrition practitioners, so you may see credentials like LD (licensed dietitian) or LN (licensed nutritionist). You can find an RD by contacting the ADA (see Appendix A for contact information). Your health care provider or local hospital may also be able to recommend an RD in your area.

FACT

According to the ADA, requirements for being an RD include a minimum of a bachelor's degree from an accredited college or university and an accredited preprofessional experience program. RDs must successfully complete a rigorous professional-level exam and must maintain ongoing continuing education to maintain their credential. Some RDs hold advanced degrees and additional certifications in specialized areas of practice.

Folic Acid and Vitamin B$_{12}$

Folic acid (folate) and vitamin B$_{12}$ are two important vitamins to be aware of even before you become pregnant. Folic acid is an issue for all women contemplating pregnancy. Since vegans must get vitamin B$_{12}$ from fortified foods or supplements, it's important to make sure that you are choosing foods or a vitamin pill that provide this essential nutrient.

Folic acid significantly lowers your baby's risk of developing neural tube defects (birth defects of the brain and spinal cord, such as spina bifida and anencephaly). Because the neural tube forms during the first four weeks of pregnancy, before many women even realize they are pregnant, the U.S. Centers for Disease Control (CDC) recommends that *all* women of childbearing age do one of the following:

❑ Take a vitamin that has folic acid in it every day. This can either be a folic acid supplement or a multivitamin. Most multivitamins sold in the United States have 400 micrograms of folic acid, the amount women need each day. Check the label of the vitamin to make sure that it contains 100 percent of the daily value (DV) of folic acid.

❑ Eat a bowl of breakfast cereal that has 100 percent of the DV of folic acid every day. Check the label on the side of the cereal box for one that has 100 percent next to folic acid.

Use of a vitamin or a breakfast cereal containing 100 percent of the DV for folic acid should be a daily practice throughout pregnancy. In addition, you can get some folic acid from other foods that you eat. Folic acid is added to breads, cereal, pasta, rice, and flour and is found naturally in leafy dark-green vegetables, citrus fruits and juices, and beans. Because the amounts in foods vary and it may be hard to get all of the folic acid you need from food sources alone, you should use either a supplement or a fortified breakfast cereal daily.

FACT

Each year, approximately 3,000 babies are born with neural tube defects. Up to 70 percent of these defects could be prevented by adequate intake of folic acid, yet according to a 2009 March of Dimes survey, less than 40 percent of American women of childbearing age (ages eighteen to forty-five) take a daily multivitamin containing folic acid to ensure they meet the daily requirements.

Vitamin B_{12} plays an important role in the development of the baby's brain and nervous system. Vegans must get vitamin B_{12} from foods fortified with this nutrient or from supplements containing vitamin B_{12}. Foods that may be fortified with vitamin B_{12} include:

- Soymilk, rice milk, and other commercial plant milks
- Meat analogs (veggie "meats")
- Breakfast cereals
- Nutritional yeast

Since vitamin B_{12} plays such an important role in the baby's development (as well as being important for your health), making sure you are accustomed to using a daily, reliable source of vitamin B_{12} before becoming pregnant is a smart, caring idea. Before you are pregnant, you need 2.4 micrograms of vitamin B_{12} daily; once you're pregnant, the amount increases to 2.6 micrograms. A food or supplement that contains at least 45 percent of the DV for vitamin B_{12} will provide enough to meet these needs.

Remember, you only need small amounts of both folic acid and vitamin B_{12}, but they are both essential vitamins. One easy way to make sure you're getting enough is to take a daily multivitamin that provides 100 percent of the DV for folic acid and at least 45 percent of the DV for vitamin B_{12}.

ALERT

Some websites claim there are nonanimal sources of vitamin B_{12} besides fortified foods or supplements. Miso, shiitake mushrooms, tempeh, sourdough bread, and umeboshi plums have all been proposed as good sources of vitamin B_{12}. When tested, however, these foods are not reliable sources. Your baby's health is too important—choose reliable fortified foods or supplements as your vitamin B_{12} sources.

Finding a Health Care Provider

Even if you have a model pregnancy, you will be seeing a lot of your health care provider over the next nine months. ACOG recommends that women see their provider every four weeks through the first twenty-eight weeks of pregnancy (about the first seven months). After week twenty-eight, the visits will increase to once every two to three weeks until week thirty-six, after which you'll be paying your doctor or midwife a weekly visit until your baby arrives. If you have any conditions that put you in a high-risk category (diabetes, history of preterm labor), your provider may want to see you more frequently to monitor your progress.

The Options

So who should guide you on this odyssey? If you currently see a gynecologist or family practice doctor who also has an obstetric practice, she may be a good choice. If you don't have that choice or would like to explore your options, consider:

- **An ob-gyn:** An obstetrician and gynecologist is a medical doctor (MD) who has received specialized training in women's health and reproductive medicine.
- **A perinatologist:** If you have a chronic health condition, you may see a perinatologist—an ob-gyn who specializes in overseeing high-risk pregnancies.
- **A midwife:** Certified nurse-midwives are licensed to practice in all fifty states. They provide patient-focused care throughout pregnancy, labor, and delivery.
- **Nurse practitioner:** A nurse practitioner (NP) is a registered nurse (RN) with advanced medical education and training (at minimum, a master's degree).
- **Combined practice:** Some obstetrical practices blend midwives, NPs, and MDs, with the choice (or sometimes the requirement) of seeing one or more of these throughout your pregnancy.

Networking and Referrals

Finding Dr. Right may seem like a monumental task. After all, this is the person you're entrusting your pregnancy and childbirth to. Unless you're paying completely out of pocket for all prenatal care, labor, and delivery expenses, your first consideration is probably your health insurance coverage. If you are part of a managed-care organization, your insurer may require that you see someone within its provider network. Getting a current copy of the network directory, if one is available, can help you narrow down your choices by coverage and location.

Need a referral? The ACOG can help you find a physician in your area (all ACOG fellows are board-certified ob-gyns). To find a nurse-midwife, contact the American College of Nurse-Midwives. (See Appendix A for contact information for both of these organizations.)

Many women choose a physician solely for logistical reasons (for example, insurance will cover all of his fees or she's near your place of work). Although money and convenience are important factors, these won't mean much if you aren't happy with the care you receive and the role they ultimately play in your pregnancy and birth. Whether your first or your fifth, this pregnancy is a one-time-only event—you deserve the best support in seeing it through. Talk to the experts—girlfriends and other women you know and trust—and get referrals. Be aware, of course, that not everyone looks for the same thing in a health care provider; what one woman emphasizes, you may downplay.

If you've just moved to a new area or simply don't know any moms or moms-to-be, there are other referral options available. The licensing authority in your area (the state or county medical board) can typically provide you with references for local practitioners. You may also try the patient services department or labor and delivery programs of nearby hospitals and/or birthing centers. Most medical centers will be happy to offer you several provider referrals, and you can get information on their facilities in the process. If you're especially interested in finding a vegan-friendly health care provider, contact local vegetarian or vegan groups to find out if others are aware of local practitioners.

Ask the Right Questions

Once you've collected names and phone numbers, narrowed down your list of potential providers, and verified that they accept (and are accepted by) your health insurance plan, it's time to do some legwork. Sit down with your partner and talk about your biggest questions, concerns, and expectations. Then compile a list of provider *interview questions*. Some issues to consider:

❑ **What are the costs and payment options?** If your health plan doesn't provide full coverage, find out how much the remaining fees will run and whether installment plans are available.

❑ **Who will deliver my baby?** Will the doctor or midwife you select deliver your child or another provider in the practice, depending on when the baby arrives? If your provider works alone, find out who covers his patients during vacations and emergencies.

❑ **Whom will I see during office visits?** Since group practices typically share delivery responsibilities, you might want to ask about rotating your prenatal appointments among all the providers in the group so you'll see a familiar face in the delivery room when the big day arrives.

❑ **What is your philosophy on routine IVs, episiotomies, labor induction, pain relief, and other interventions in the birth process?** If you have certain expectations regarding medical interventions during labor and delivery, you should lay them out now.

❑ **What hospital or birthing center will I go to?** Find out where the provider has hospital privileges and obtain more information on that facility's programs and policies, if possible. Is a neonatal unit available if problems arise after the baby's birth? Many hospitals offer tours of their labor and delivery rooms for expectant parents.

❑ **What is your policy on birth plans?** Will the provider work with you to create and, more important, to follow a birth plan? Will the plan be signed, and become part of your permanent chart in case she is off duty during the birth? (For more on birth plans, see Chapter 15 and Appendix B.)

❑ **How are phone calls handled if I have a health concern or question?** Most obstetrical practices have some sort of triage (or prioritizing) system in place for patient phone calls. Ask how quickly calls are returned and what system the practice has in place for handling night and weekend patient calls.

Some providers have the staff to answer these sorts of inquiries over the phone, while others might schedule a face-to-face appointment with your prospective doctor or midwife. Either way, make sure that all your questions are answered to your satisfaction so you can make a fully informed choice.

Comfort and Communication

As with any good relationship, communication is essential between patients and their providers. Does the provider encourage your questions, answer them thoroughly, and really listen to your concerns? Does he make sure all your questions are answered before concluding the appointment? Are the nursing and administrative staff attentive to patients' needs and willing to answer questions as well?

Good health care is a partnership or, more accurately, a team effort. Although ultimately you call the shots (it's your body and your baby, after all), your provider serves as your coach and trainer, giving you the support and training you need to reach the finish line. If your doctor doesn't listen to your needs in the first place, she won't be able to meet them. Remember as well that communication works both ways. Your provider has likely been around the block a few times and has a wealth of useful information to offer you, particularly if you're a rookie at this baby game.

Gender may also be an issue for you. Some women feel more at ease with a female physician because of communication style and the fact that the physician may have been through pregnancy herself. Other women prefer a male doctor for various reasons. Making an issue of gender may seem silly or, at worst, discriminatory and hypocritical. The subject is serious enough to merit a number of clinical studies and patient surveys in the medical literature both for and against a clear gender preference. The bottom line is that you are the one who has to live with your provider choice for the next nine months, and to spend it feeling awkward, stressed, and inhibited—emotions that can ultimately have a negative effect on your pregnancy—is not healthy. Whatever your choice, make sure it's one you'll be comfortable with.

Talking to Your Health Care Provider about Your Vegan Diet

You may be fortunate enough to find a health care provider who is either vegan or very knowledgeable about vegan diets. If so, consider yourself lucky. It's more likely that your practitioner has, at best, a passing knowledge of vegan diets, perhaps gleaned from an article she read years ago. This is a great opportunity to educate your provider so that you can work together to ensure a healthy pregnancy.

You may wonder if you should even mention your vegan diet at all. In the spirit of open communication and honesty, you should. Saying something like, "I've been vegan for the past five years and feel pretty comfortable with my diet," lets your doctor know that you've been doing this for a while and that you're confident about your choice. If you've worked with an RD (or plan to do so), mention this.

Your health care provider may smile, say something positive, "Great! Thanks for letting me know. Some of my healthiest patients are vegans," and move on. He may ask you for more details like which foods you avoid or where you get various nutrients. Come prepared (but not defensive). Describe your diet in simple, positive terms: "I eat beans, whole grains, nuts, fruits, and vegetables. I don't eat meat, fish, poultry, eggs, or dairy products." Think about where you get some key nutrients like protein, vitamin B_{12}, calcium, iron, and vitamin D (see upcoming chapters for details) and be ready to answer questions. This could be an opportunity to fine-tune your dietary choices as you prepare for pregnancy.

If you'd like to go a bit farther, give your health care provider a brief update on vegan diets: "I recently read that the American Dietetic Association said well-planned vegan diets were fine for pregnant women." Offer to share references. Provide your doctor with a link to the ADA's position paper on vegetarian diets (see Appendix A) or other resources. Bring in this book and share it with your doctor. By keeping the tone positive, upbeat, and informational, you're letting your provider know that you're willing to work as a partner and that you're knowledgeable about your diet.

If, despite your best efforts, your potential provider continues to disparage vegan diets, it may be time to courteously end the visit and consider whether or not this is the right provider for you.

Exercising Your Body

Women often wonder whether or not they should start, stop, increase, or decrease their exercise routines if they're trying to get pregnant. In most cases, regular exercise before getting pregnant is encouraged. Plenty of exercise promotes good health throughout your life. Exercise can help you lose a few pounds if you need to before becoming pregnant. Your ability to stay active throughout your pregnancy depends on your health and activity level before pregnancy.

If you're just starting out with exercising, start with something simple like walking, swimming, or biking. If you are not used to a lot of exercise, check with your doctor about safety guidelines and don't overdo at first. Gradually increase both the time and intensity of your exercise.

Smoking Cessation

You don't need anyone to tell you that cigarettes are bad for you. If you are a smoker, you've probably tried to stop, possibly more than once. It's not an easy endeavor, but now that you're contemplating pregnancy, you have special motivation to quit and make it stick. Smoking exposes you to health risks such as cardiovascular disease, lung cancer, and high blood pressure; it can also have dire consequences for your baby.

According to the U.S. Surgeon General, women who smoke place their child at increased risk for premature birth and stillbirth as well as prenatal complications such as premature rupture of membranes (PROM), placenta previa, placental abruption, and intrauterine growth restriction (IUGR). The dangers continue after birth, with an increased risk of sudden infant death syndrome (SIDS), low birth weight, recurrent ear infections, and of later development of psychosocial problems such as conduct disorder and substance abuse. Even environmental exposure to tobacco smoke can be detrimental; secondhand smoke causes a slightly increased risk of both IUGR and low birth weight. Encourage your partner to stop smoking as well, since living with secondhand smoke can be harmful to you and your baby. Cigarettes also take a toll on the pocketbook; neonatal care costs attributable to smoking account for over $360 million annually.

If you're a smoker, ideally, you will kick the habit in the planning stages of your pregnancy. Even if you're pregnant and still smoking, quitting now can make a big difference to your baby's health. Women who stop smoking in the first trimester of pregnancy greatly reduce the risk of IUGR for their child.

Using Medications

Medication use in pregnancy is a thorny issue. There is simply not enough long-term clinical data available on most drugs to provide a 100 percent guarantee of their safety. Ideally, you should avoid all prescription and over-the-counter drugs, except for your prenatal supplements, throughout pregnancy. However, that's an unrealistic expectation given that up to 64 percent of all pregnant women take one or more prescription drugs at some point in their pregnancy. And if you have a chronic disease, such as diabetes, schizophrenia, or HIV, you have little choice but to continue your treatment.

The FDA has a classification system for drugs based on the degree of known risk a medication presents to a fetus. The following chart outlines the five categories currently used for establishing drug safety in pregnancy:

Category	Description
A	Adequate, well-controlled studies in pregnant women have not shown an increased risk of fetal abnormalities.
B	Animal studies have revealed no evidence of harm to the fetus; however, there are no adequate and well-controlled studies in pregnant women. OR: Animal studies have shown an adverse effect, but adequate and well-controlled studies in pregnant women have failed to demonstrate a risk to the fetus.
C	Animal studies have shown an adverse effect, and there are no adequate and well-controlled studies in pregnant women. OR: No animal studies have been conducted, and there are no adequate and well-controlled studies in pregnant women.
D	Adequate, well-controlled, or observational studies in pregnant women have demonstrated a risk to the fetus. However, the benefits of therapy may outweigh the potential risk.
X	Adequate, well-controlled, or observational studies in animals or pregnant women have demonstrated positive evidence of fetal abnormalities. The use of the product is contraindicated, or not advised, in women who are or may become pregnant.

The consequences of not taking a medication must also be taken into consideration when evaluating the use of a drug. Do the benefits of the drug outweigh the risks to the mother and/or fetus? Can a safer medication be substituted temporarily? Or can the drug be temporarily stopped during the period of time it is known to potentially harm the fetus? With close observation, well-researched prescribing, and careful dosing, the use of medication can proceed safely in many cases. It's good to discuss these issues with your health care provider when you're thinking about getting pregnant. That way you can plan the best way to proceed.

There are a number of drugs that are teratogens—meaning that they have been shown to cause birth defects or other developmental problems in pregnancy. Following is a partial list of some well-known offenders. This list is not all-inclusive, and you should discuss all medication use with your practitioner.

- Angiotensin converting enzyme inhibitors (ACE inhibitors; prescribed for high blood pressure)
- Accutane (isotretinoin; prescribed for cystic acne)
- Androgens (testosterone, danazol; prescribed for endometriosis)

- Anticonvulsants (prescribed for seizure disorders or irregular heartbeats)
- Atypical antipsychotics (prescribed for schizophrenia and bipolar disorder; linked to risk of neural tube defects)
- Certain antibiotics (including streptomycin and tetracycline)
- Certain anticoagulants (warfarin; to prevent blood clotting)
- Tapazole (methimazole; an antithyroid drug prescribed for hyperthyroidism)
- Aspirin and nonsteroidal anti-inflammatory drugs (NSAIDs; for pain relief) during the last trimester
- Chemotherapeutic drugs (used to treat cancer and skin diseases)
- Diethylstilbestrol (DES; not prescribed for pregnant women after the Food and Drug Administration issued a warning in 1971)
- Lithium (used for treatment of depression and bipolar disorder)
- Thalidomide (prescribed for leprosy and inflammatory conditions; in limited use due to its high potential for causing birth defects)

Sometimes women decide to self-treat colds and other illnesses with dietary supplements and herbal and botanical remedies before and during pregnancy, mistakenly assuming that medicine from a botanical source is inherently safe for their fetus. Remember: *Natural* doesn't necessarily mean harmless; herbs can be potent medicinal substances. Even seemingly benign substances like herbal tea have the potential to interact with other foods and medications and cause harm to your developing child. Since you may not be aware that you are pregnant for the first few weeks, if there is a possibility that you could be pregnant, always check with your care provider before taking anything medicinal, herbal or otherwise.

Avoiding Alcohol

So what about alcohol? You may have heard that moderate consumption of a drink or two a week is safe in pregnancy. The truth is that *there is absolutely no known safe level of alcohol intake in pregnancy,* and even a single beer or glass of wine may have an impact on the development of your unborn child. Bottom line—complete abstinence is the safest route for baby. Even if you're not pregnant, if you're thinking about having a baby, now is the time to get a handle on even occasional drinking, not to mention binge or frequent drinking. If you're concerned about your drinking habits, talk to your health care provider about treatment options or turn to your place of worship or local social service agency for support.

Suppose that, as you read this, you are pregnant already and realize that you have had a cocktail since conception, perhaps before you even discovered you were pregnant. There is no point in obsessing over that drink. Letting the incident consume you with guilt or allowing it to become a source of undue stress is bad for you and baby. Instead, focus your energies on following a healthy lifestyle now.

FACT

The CDC estimates that approximately one in every 1,000 live births results in fetal alcohol syndrome, at a cost of approximately $4 billion annually. Although there are no official statistics on fetal alcohol spectrum disorders, it is estimated that they occur three times as often as fetal alcohol syndrome.

The consequences of continuing alcohol use during pregnancy range from risking miscarriage to causing an array of physical, mental, behavioral, and developmental problems known as fetal alcohol spectrum disorders (FASD). One of the most severe is fetal alcohol syndrome (FAS). Babies born with FAS experience growth retardation, central nervous system problems, as well as develop characteristic facial features including small eye openings; a small head; a short, upturned nose; absence of the groove between the upper lip and the nose; and an undeveloped outer ear. FAS is permanent and irreversible.

Since the first eight weeks of pregnancy are a time of rapid development for the limbs, heart, central nervous system, and other organ systems of the embryo, it's important to avoid alcohol to reduce the risk of problems for your baby. Talk to your partner also. Some studies have found that if your partner drinks, smokes, or uses drugs, it can lower his fertility and possibly damage his sperm.

CHAPTER 3

Vegan Nutrition: Protein

What nutrition question are vegans asked most often? If you guessed, "Where do you get protein?" or something similar, you're probably right. People mistakenly believe that you can only get enough protein from a diet heavy on beef, pork, chicken, fish, dairy products, and eggs with added protein powder "just to be sure." Not to worry. Most people, vegans included, get plenty of protein, even when their protein needs are higher because of strenuous exercise or, more relevantly, being pregnant.

Protein Needs

The word "protein" comes from the Greek word *proteios*, meaning "primary." Perhaps this word was chosen because of protein's primary role in body function. Proteins are responsible for everything from the structure of your muscles and bones to the proper function of your immune system to food digestion. Many hormones are made from protein. Adequate protein is needed for healthy skin, hair, and nails. In pregnancy, extra protein is needed to support your baby's growth—building bones and muscles, for example. You also need extra protein as your blood volume increases and your breasts and uterus enlarge.

FACT

During pregnancy, you'll gain a bit more than 2 pounds of protein. About a pound of this is accounted for by your baby's muscle, hair, skin, bones, teeth, and internal organs. The other pound or so is added to your usual body protein content.

Before you were pregnant, you needed around 0.4 grams of protein for every pound that you weighed. The math isn't hard to do. Take your prepregnant weight in pounds and multiply by 0.4—that's how much protein you needed before you were pregnant. For instance, if you weighed 120 pounds, you'd multiply 120 by 0.4 (calculators allowed, this is not a test) and get 48 grams of protein. The first trimester of pregnancy, you actually don't need any more protein than this because your baby is so small and your body changes are less than they will be later on.

Protein Needs in the Second and Third Trimesters

Starting with the fourth month of pregnancy, protein needs increase to support changes to your body and your baby's growth. You need about 25 grams of protein a day more than you did before you were pregnant or in the first trimester. Simply take the amount of protein recommended before pregnancy (0.4 times your prepregnant weight) and add 25. That's how much daily protein (in grams) is recommended. This amount is about 50 percent higher than protein recommendations for nonpregnant women. So for instance, if you weighed 120 pounds before pregnancy, you'd multiply 120 by 0.4 and then add 25 for a total of 73 grams of protein.

QUESTION

Do vegans need more protein than meat eaters?
Some vegan nutrition experts recommend that vegans get slightly more protein than nonvegans. Their rationale is that vegan protein sources like beans and whole grains are harder to digest. They suggest about 10 percent more protein for vegans. This amount is pretty small and is nothing to be concerned about. If you want to calculate, multiply your protein recommendation by 1.1.

If you're lucky enough to be expecting twins, you'll need extra protein. After all, instead of one baby, you have two on the way. Moms of twins should add 50 grams of protein to their prepregnant protein needs. So, if you calculated your protein needs before you were pregnant as 48 grams a day, you'd add 50 grams for a total of 98 grams of protein to aim for in the second and third trimesters.

Vegan Protein Sources

The list of vegan foods that don't contain protein is a much shorter list than those foods that do supply protein. Foods that provide protein include all varieties of beans from adzuki to yellow beans, grains, nuts and seeds, nut butters and seed butters, vegetables, potatoes, soy foods, meat analogs (products made to resemble meats), and seitan (wheat "meat"). The short list of poor sources of protein is just that, short.

Foods and ingredients that are not good sources of protein include:

- Fats and oils—margarine, olive oil, canola oil, other oils, most salad dressings
- Sugar and other sweeteners like maple syrup, molasses, and agave nectar
- Soft drinks, coffee, tea

- Herbs and spices—the amounts you eat are too small to provide much protein
- Fruits. Note that fruits are great foods—they're just not good protein sources
- Alcohol (But you're not drinking that anyway, right?)

So unless you're feasting on hard candy, fried bananas, wine coolers, and the like for every meal, every day, chances are that you're getting a good amount of protein.

When you go for a routine prenatal visit to your doctor, your urine will be tested for protein. This is mainly a test for preeclampsia, urinary tract infection, and kidney function. This test does not provide information about how much protein is in your diet.

The other thing to be aware of is getting enough calories. Ideally, you're gaining weight at the rate that you should for pregnancy. If you are, chances are that you're getting enough calories. Not gaining weight could mean fewer calories than you need, which means that protein is being used mainly to keep your body functions going instead of being used to build your baby's muscles.

Your protein intake will naturally increase as you eat more food when you are pregnant, especially if you focus on foods that are good sources of protein.

How Much Protein Are You Eating?

You're probably not going to approach each meal with a calculator in hand to make sure that you're meeting your protein needs. Chances are you don't even need to be concerned about protein. An occasional spot check, however, can provide peace of mind. Here's how to do it. First, write down everything you eat for a typical day and how much you ate of each food. Then, use an online nutrition program to calculate how much protein you ate. One recommended website is *www.mypyramidtracker.gov*. While this website's database does contain information about thousands of foods, it may not include many vegan foods that you are familiar with. Use food labels to see how much protein is in foods that aren't in the database. Refer to recommendations in this chapter for protein intake in pregnancy; this website's recommendations have not been modified for pregnancy. Compare your protein needs to the amount of protein in your diet and make any adjustments needed.

Remember, this is just one day. If you eat much the same from one day to the next, you can be pretty confident that your results provide a reliable picture of your diet. If your eating habits vary widely, make sure that your diet has several good sources of protein every day.

Protein in Vegan Foods

Some vegan foods that are especially high in protein are soybeans, tempeh, and lentils. These foods have 20 or more grams of protein in a serving—a cup of beans or 4 ounces of tempeh. Other foods that provide generous amounts of protein (10–20 grams per serving) include tofu, veggie burgers, and cooked dried beans. Soymilk, peanut butter, soy yogurt, and quinoa are all good sources of protein as well. Vegetables, whole grains, pasta, almond butter, and nuts and seeds are other good foods to add to your protein intake.

There are some easy ways to incorporate good sources of protein into your daily meal plan. These are all highly nutritious foods, so by adding them you're not just adding protein but a host of vitamins and minerals as well.

AT BREAKFAST
- Spread some peanut butter or other nut butter on your toast or bagel; peanut butter can even top oatmeal—add a spoonful of jelly for PB and J oatmeal.
- Blend soft or silken tofu with soymilk and fruit (fresh, frozen, or canned) for a quick smoothie. See Chapter 17 for more smoothie ideas.
- Use soymilk in place of water to prepare hot cereals.
- Mix things up with a bowl of quinoa instead of oatmeal.
- Replace water or other liquids in your favorite muffin and pancake recipes with soymilk.
- On more leisurely mornings, try a tofu scramble or quiche for breakfast. See Chapter 17 for recipe ideas.

AT LUNCH

- Toss some chickpeas or black beans with your salad.
- Use a flavored hummus in place of mayo as a savory sandwich spread.
- Prepare a vegan cream soup with soymilk.
- Add extra crunch to a peanut butter sandwich by sprinkling on coarsely chopped peanuts or other nuts.
- Pack protein-rich leftovers to reheat at lunchtime.

AT DINNER

- Purée white beans or soft tofu with your favorite tomato sauce and serve over whole-grain pasta.
- Top baked potatoes with a spoonful of plain soy yogurt and some chopped chives.
- A peanut sauce (homemade or purchased) can top rice, pasta, or vegetables.
- Add chickpeas or vegan pepperoni to takeout or homemade veggie no-cheese pizza.
- Experiment with quinoa in dishes that use rice or other grains.
- Toss vegan stir-fry strips or homemade seitan with stir-fried vegetables.

FOR SNACKS

- Make a batch of trail mix using a variety of nuts and dried fruits. Add soy nuts for a protein boost.
- Spread apple or pear slices with nut butters.
- Dip baby carrots and jicama strips into hummus or refried beans.
- Try different brands of vegan energy bars until you find one or more that suit you.
- Eat breakfast for a snack by having a bowl of cold cereal with soymilk.

If you like to bake, you can boost the protein in breads and muffins by adding soy flour. For yeast-raised breads, put 2 tablespoons of soy flour in your 1 cup measuring cup and then fill the cup with the flour your recipe calls for. Repeat until you've measured all of the recipe's flour. Since soy flour does not contain gluten, which gives bread its structure, it cannot completely replace wheat flour. For quick breads or muffins, replace up to a quarter of the flour with soy flour.

You'll probably think of even more ways to add protein-rich soy products, beans, seitan, nuts, and nut butters to your meals and snacks.

Protein Combining

Have you ever been asked if you "combine" proteins? Many years ago, a popular book called *Diet for a Small Planet* promoted vegetarian diets and the idea of eating certain foods together to make sure people met their protein needs. For example, beans were to be eaten with rice, and peanut butter with whole grains. While *Diet for a Small Planet* succeeded in making vegetarian eating seem safe and possible, it also made people think it was much more complicated to be vegetarian than it really is. Imagine having to precisely measure the amount of beans on your plate and then decide exactly how much rice you had to eat to "complement" the beans!

Protein combining is based on the fact that humans need certain amino acids in order to build each type of protein. For example, the protein found in your hair would use a different mixture of amino acids than the protein found in your muscles. Fortunately, your body is able to store amino acids from one meal to the next, so it's not necessary to eat perfect amounts of amino acids at every meal.

There are nine amino acids your body cannot make, so you have to get them from foods. Some vegan foods contain generous amounts of all nine essential amino acids. These foods include soy products (soybeans, tofu, tempeh, and soymilk), quinoa, and hemp seed. Other foods still provide some of each essential amino acid; they may be higher in one and lower in another compared to the so-called reference proteins (like cow's milk and eggs).

By eating a variety of foods over the entire day, you can eliminate the need to worry about strict protein combining. The higher levels of the amino acid lysine in the bean dip you eat for a snack will supplement breakfast's whole-wheat toast that doesn't have that much lysine. In turn, the whole-wheat toast can provide a boost in methionine, an amino acid that is lower in beans. Experienced vegans don't even think about protein combining. They simply eat a variety of good sources of protein like beans, grains, nuts, and soy products over the course of the day.

Food Cravings

Some vegan moms-to-be report protein cravings. All of a sudden, a committed vegan is craving steak or broiled salmon. If this happens to you, you may wonder if it indicates a dietary deficiency. Chances are good that it doesn't. Scientists don't really understand why some people experience cravings for certain foods, but studies have shown that the food being craved has no relationship to nutritional status.

So how do you explain the craving for a juicy burger or a wedge of cheese? It may simply be that you've been conditioned to equate protein, especially meat or dairy products, with health. In pregnancy, when you're trying to do everything right for your baby, those old habits kick in and you may question whether or not you're getting what you need. Step back and look at what you are eating. It may even be worthwhile in terms of peace of mind to make an appointment with an RD who is knowledgeable about vegan nutrition. He can look at your eating habits and let you know if you need to make any adjustments to get enough protein on your vegan diet. Chances are that you won't need to make changes, but it is reassuring to have another set of eyes look at what you're eating.

Cravings may also be for comfort, rather than food. When you're dreaming of your mom's meatloaf, maybe you're really longing for the good old days when your biggest responsibility was walking the dog or setting the table. If that's the case, try some alternative comfort measures instead of Mom's meatloaf recipe. Order a vegan take-out meal, soak in a hot tub, or call a friend.

Some women find that eating a vegan meat look-alike helps them cope with their cravings. Others report success with eating something salty or a bit fatty, a handful of salted nuts or a spoonful of hummus, for instance.

Food cravings, and not just for higher protein foods, are common in pregnancy. Whether it's the stereotypical pickles and ice cream or something else, you may find yourself really wanting a certain food, not necessarily something you would usually eat. Some researchers believe that these kinds of cravings are due to hormonal changes that accompany pregnancy. These hormone shifts lead to an intensified sense of smell. Since smell is related to taste, there may be some connection between smells, tastes, and cravings. You may find that your cravings change from day to day and even from one pregnancy to the next.

You may find yourself craving fresh fruit or vegetables. If that's the case, keep the refrigerator stocked with these healthy snacks. If, however, you find that your cravings are leading to frequent junk food binges, it's time for some coping tips.

- Low blood sugar may trigger cravings. Try to avoid precipitous drops in your blood sugar levels by eating small frequent meals and snacks.
- Emotional stress may also play a role. Ask yourself if this is really a craving or a reaction to stress or boredom. Think of coping mechanisms like taking a walk or doing some gentle yoga.
- Sometimes a craving can be satisfied by eating a bite or two of the food you're fixated on. Eat a bite and then do something else. And don't leave the open bag of chips on the counter!
- Try to think of a healthier substitute for the food you crave. If you're craving French fries, make oven-baked fries; instead of a pound bag of chocolate chips, try a cup of hot cocoa.

Cravings will pass with time. It's unlikely that after your baby is born you'll still be longing for peanut butter and barbecue potato chip sandwiches!

Protein Myths

Myths about protein abound. From rumors that unless you eat meat you're in danger of protein deficiency to the mistaken notion that proteins have to be carefully combined, there is a lot of misinformation about protein. Hopefully, you're already convinced that protein adequacy is entirely possible on a vegan diet and that careful meal-based protein combining is not necessary. There are other myths about protein that you may encounter.

Plant Proteins Are Incomplete

This myth, that plant proteins are incomplete, or somehow inferior to animal proteins, refers to the amino acids in plant proteins. While protein from plants contains all of the nine essential amino acids, some amino acids may be present in lower amounts in plant proteins than in animal-derived protein. Eating a variety of plant protein sources makes it likely, however, that you'll get the amount of amino acids that you need.

Vegans Need to Use Protein Supplements

Protein supplements come in different forms, most commonly powders that are mixed with water or other liquids. Vegan protein supplements do exist and are usually based on soy, rice, or hemp protein. If you are eating a varied vegan diet that includes good sources of protein, it's unlikely that any protein supplement is needed. Of course, if you have a number of food restrictions because of allergies or intolerances or have especially high protein needs because of a medical condition, your RD may suggest using protein supplements. For most vegan women, however, they are an unnecessary expense.

Exercising Markedly Increases Your Protein Needs

The area of protein needs with strenuous exercise is a controversial one. Some research suggests that people engaging in strenuous exercise have somewhat higher protein needs while other research does not support any increase in protein. The kind of strenuous exercise that might affect protein needs is not the kind that you are doing while pregnant. Protein needs are higher for those who are training for a fast-paced marathon or doing intensive weight lifting for body building purposes. Your protein needs are already somewhat higher in the second and third trimesters of your pregnancy; the exercise you participate in during pregnancy—walking, biking, swimming, or even running—should not be strenuous enough to markedly increase your protein needs above those of pregnancy.

Vegan Etiquette: When Others Ask about Protein

You're at a restaurant with your coworkers and someone remembers that you're vegan. They also know you're pregnant. With a concerned look, they ask, "Now that you're pregnant, how are you going to be able to get enough protein on a vegan diet?" Remember, it's likely that:

- They are genuinely concerned
- They know next to nothing about vegan nutrition

- Their eyes will start to glaze over if your answer takes more than a minute or two
- They really want reassurance that you're on top of things and aren't doing anything harmful

Keep your answer brief, calm, friendly, and positive. Even if you've answered this question hundreds of times, simply say something like, "I've been reading some excellent books about vegan nutrition just to make sure I'm doing everything right. I get the protein I need from beans, grains, soy products, nuts, and vegetables." And then change the subject, "I'm having the veggie burger with a baked potato. How about you?"

CHAPTER 4

Vegan Nutrition: Iron and Zinc

The requirements for iron and zinc are very small (think milligrams), but these minerals play important roles in your baby's development. Vegans face the challenge of compensating for reduced absorption of iron and zinc from plant foods. On the positive side, plants also contain absorption-boosting substances. Many women will be advised by their health care provider to take iron pills during pregnancy because it is so challenging for most women (not just vegans) to get enough iron solely from food at this time of high iron needs.

Iron Needs

Iron's major role is to help red blood cells deliver oxygen throughout your body. When you are pregnant, iron also helps deliver oxygen to your baby. Women's need for iron increases dramatically in pregnancy, especially in the second and third trimesters. In pregnancy, your body's blood supply actually increases 40–50 percent. In order to make this extra blood, you need more iron than you do when you're not pregnant. Your unborn baby is also storing iron that will last for the first few months of life outside your womb. Baby takes what she needs from your store of iron first, so she won't suffer unless you are very low in iron. However, you can end up with iron-deficiency anemia.

After your baby is born, your iron needs go down dramatically. Not only are you not making extra blood or supporting your baby's growth anymore, but you also won't be having menstrual periods for a little while, which means you're not losing iron each month in menstrual flow.

Pregnancy does boost the amount of iron that you absorb, especially in the second trimester. Eating foods that contain plenty of iron lets you take advantage of this natural increase in iron absorption. Nonvegetarians don't benefit as much from the increased iron absorption later in pregnancy, since only the nonheme form of iron is better absorbed.

Iron for Vegans

Recommendations for iron are higher for vegetarians than for nonvegetarians. This is because all of the iron in vegetarian diets is found in a form called nonheme iron, which is not as well absorbed as some of the iron found in meat. Part of the iron in meat is in a form called heme iron, which is especially well absorbed.

When you consider that vegan diets can be particularly high in substances that interfere with iron absorption, you can see why the Institute of Medicine (the folks who create nutrient recommendations) suggests that vegetarians need 1.8 times more iron than nonvegetarians.

That's not to say, of course, that you can't get the iron you need on a vegetarian diet. It's possible, with smart food choices, for vegan women to meet the vegetarian Recommended Dietary Allowance (RDA) for nonpregnant women of 32 milligrams of iron per day. When you add in the higher iron needs that go with pregnancy, however, many women find that taking a daily iron pill, along with choosing high iron foods, is what they need. Depending on the amount of iron in your diet and the amount of iron in your prenatal vitamin-mineral supplement, you may not need to take additional iron. That's something that you can discuss with your health care provider, who will make recommendations based on the iron levels in your blood and your food choices.

Vegan Iron Sources

Even if you are taking an iron pill or getting most of the iron you need from your prenatal supplement, it still makes sense to choose foods high in iron. Why? These foods aren't just iron powerhouses; many of them are the basis for a healthy vegan diet because they are such good sources of other nutrients.

ESSENTIAL

Some foods have extra iron added. Two that come to mind are some brands of breakfast cereals and some veggie "meats." If you're looking for high-iron foods, check the Nutrition Facts label. If iron is added you'll see larger numbers like 30 percent, 60 percent, or 100 percent in the iron row.

You've heard of some of these foods in earlier chapters—dried beans, soy products, leafy green veggies, whole grains. Others may be less familiar. Did you know that a tablespoon of blackstrap molasses has more iron than ½ cup of spinach? Sea vegetables are another, possibly less familiar, iron source.

Making Good Choices: Breads and Cereals

Whole grains—foods like whole-wheat flour, brown rice, and oatmeal—have undergone minimal processing. These foods and other whole grains are good sources of iron. When grains are refined (think white flour, white rice, and degermed cornmeal), the part of the grain that contains the most iron is removed. Sure, this improves shelf life and, if you like white, makes for a more attractive product, but it also reduces the nutritional quality of the grain. In order to compensate for this, refined grains often have some nutrients added back, including iron. This means that both whole grains and enriched grains (refined grains that have some nutrients added back) are good sources of iron.

Another grain source of iron is wheat germ. Wheat germ is the high iron part of wheat that is removed when wheat is refined. By adding a spoonful or two of wheat germ to smoothies or hot cereal, you can boost the iron in these foods.

Making Good Choices: Beans and Soy Foods

Dried beans and soy products are foods vegans turn to in order to meet their iron needs. A cup of cooked lentils has about as much iron as three-and-a-half chicken drumsticks or a 9-ounce hamburger. All dried beans and peas are good sources of iron. Green beans, of course, are not dried beans and don't have the iron that dried beans do.

ESSENTIAL

Some great vegan sources of iron don't fit neatly into categories like dried beans, vegetables, grains, or fruits. Foods like blackstrap molasses, dark chocolate, and energy bars are easy ways to add some extra iron. Blackstrap molasses is a by-product of sugar production. It is high not just in iron, but also in calcium and other minerals.

Soy foods, based on soybeans, are also high in iron. Soybeans have more iron than other dried beans, so products made from soybeans like tofu, tempeh, and soymilk are also good sources of iron. Some veggie "meats" have extra iron added to them. Check the Nutrition Facts label to help identify these products.

Making Good Choices: Vegetables and Sea Vegetables

Vegetables vary widely in terms of their iron content. For instance, you'd have to eat 3 cups of iceberg lettuce in order to get as much iron as you would from a single cup of raw spinach. Six cups of cooked cauliflower or carrot sticks would have as much iron as 1 cup of green peas. And it would take a whopping 8 cups of sautéed mushrooms to have as much iron as 1 cup of cooked collard greens.

As a group, green vegetables are good iron sources. Green vegetables include leafy greens like spinach, beet greens, collards, kale, and Swiss chard. Other green vegetables like asparagus, Brussels sprouts, and bok choy also supply iron. Tomato products including sun-dried tomatoes, tomato juice, and tomato sauce are another way to add iron to your diet.

Sea vegetables, as the name suggests, are vegetables harvested from the sea. You may have tried nori, a sea vegetable that forms the wrapping for sushi rolls. Other sea vegetables include kombu, dulse, and wakame (pronounced *wah-ka-may*). Sea vegetables are often sold in dried form and may need to be rehydrated before using. They have a pleasant, salty-sweet taste and can be added to salads, soups, grain dishes, or stir-fries. Kombu is especially high in iron, but most sea vegetables are also excellent sources of iron and other minerals.

Making Good Choices: Fruits and Nuts

If you're looking to fruit as a way to boost your iron intake, focus on dried fruits. Dried apricots, raisins, and prunes are actually not higher in iron than their fresh counterparts; it's just that most people can eat a handful of raisins without feeling as full as they would from eating an equivalent amount of grapes. Don't forget prune juice and apricot nectar—they're also ways to add iron.

FACT

Roasted pumpkin seeds can be made at home using seeds from your Halloween jack-o-lantern. Clean the seeds, removing all pumpkin flesh and strings. Let dry. Toss with a little oil, salt, and spices. Spread in a single layer on a cookie sheet and bake at 275°F for 10–20 minutes, checking often so they don't burn.

The best iron choices from the nuts and seeds food group are cashews, pumpkin seeds, and sunflower seeds. While other nuts do supply some iron, cashews have more iron than almonds, pecans, or walnuts.

Tahini (sesame seed butter) may be familiar if you're used to making your own hummus (it's an ingredient in many recipes). It can also be stirred into grains or vegetable dishes. With close to 3 milligrams of iron in 2 table-spoons, tahini has more iron than other nut or seed butters.

Top Vegan Iron Sources

While many foods vegans eat supply iron, the following foods are some of the highest sources:

1. Iron-fortified breakfast cereals
2. Cream of Wheat or instant oatmeal
3. Tofu
4. Sea vegetables
5. Iron-fortified energy bars
6. Soybeans
7. Dark chocolate
8. Lentils
9. Spinach
10. Garbanzo beans

Menu Makeovers

Take some of your favorite vegan meals and see what changes you can make to boost their iron content. You'll probably find that you're eating healthier overall when you make these changes.

For example, if your go-to breakfast is orange juice, Shredded Wheat with strawberries and soymilk, and toast with peanut butter, try these changes:

- Swirl some prune juice in with the OJ.
- Sprinkle a spoonful of wheat germ on your cereal along with the strawberries.
- Choose a higher iron cereal—either a fortified ready-to-eat cereal or oatmeal.
- Try replacing the peanut butter with high-iron tahini and top your toast with raisins.

If you usually snack on pretzels and fruit, make an iron-rich trail mix with dried apricots, cashews, and pumpkin or sunflower seeds.

Here's a dinner makeover. If your menu features stir-fried green beans, broccoli, and carrots with almonds over brown rice:

- Replace all or part of the vegetables with higher iron choices—peas, spinach, Swiss chard, for instance.
- Season the stir-fry with nori flakes.
- Add a higher iron protein source like firm tofu cubes or some navy beans or other beans.
- In place of adding beans to the stir-fry, add another dish containing beans—maybe a hummus dip or lentil soup as an appetizer.
- Choose another grain, quinoa for example, or serve the stir-fry over enriched pasta.
- Treat yourself to a small piece of dark chocolate for dessert.

Making the Most of Dietary Iron

Nonheme iron, the only form of iron found in plants, is absorbed to a greater or lesser extent depending on the other foods that are eaten along with plant sources of iron. Substances called phytates are major inhibitors of iron absorption. Phytates are found in a number of foods vegans commonly eat including whole grains, dried beans, nuts, seeds, and vegetables. It may seem that almost every food that you think of as a good vegan iron source contains these substances that interfere with iron absorption.

The good news is that foods that provide vitamin C can pretty much counteract phytates' interfering actions. Something as simple as drinking a small glass of orange juice with a meal can increase the amount of iron absorbed as much as 400 percent, even if phytates are present.

It's not just orange juice that can help increase iron absorption. All citrus fruits and juices provide vitamin C. So do tomatoes and tomato products (tomato sauce, tomato juice, and tomato soup), broccoli, cauliflower, cabbage, cantaloupe, kiwi, pineapple, kale, sweet potatoes—most fruits and many vegetables can add vitamin C.

The trick is to have the food that provides vitamin C at the same meal as the foods high in iron. For simplicity's sake, try to have a vitamin C source at most meals—a piece of fruit, a small glass of juice, or a serving of vegetables; not only will iron absorption be improved, but you'll also be eating healthier.

Another trick for promoting iron absorption is to use more foods produced or preserved by the action of microorganisms, commonly called fermented foods. These foods like sauerkraut, traditional soy sauce, tempeh, and sourdough bread contain organic acids that promote iron absorption.

Coffee (both regular and decaffeinated), tea (including some herb teas), and cocoa contain substances that interfere with iron absorption. If you use these beverages, wait to have them until several hours have gone by after a meal with a lot of iron in it to keep substances in the beverages from blocking your body's uptake of that iron.

Calcium supplements can also interfere with iron absorption. If you're taking calcium pills, take them between meals.

Iron Deficiency

About half of all pregnant women develop iron-deficiency anemia. That's because pregnant women need twice as much iron as they usually do and because many women aren't getting enough iron even before they are pregnant. Women frequently have low amounts of iron stored in their bodies.

There's no evidence that vegan women have higher rates of iron deficiency. Because iron-deficiency anemia can increase the risk of having a premature or low birth-weight baby, it's routine to check the iron status of all pregnant women.

Anemia can make you feel weak, tired, and dizzy. So can pregnancy. A blood test is needed to help sort things out.

Iron status is commonly checked by drawing a blood sample and determining the levels of hemoglobin and hematocrit. This is typically done at your first prenatal visit. Iron status may be checked again in the second and third trimesters. Your iron status may be checked more frequently if your blood is low in iron.

If low levels are found you will probably be given iron supplements to take. Additional tests of iron status may be done. Measuring blood levels of a substance called ferritin provides an indication of how much iron you have stored in your body. Ideally, you would have some extra iron stored to replace any blood losses or to compensate for times when you're not eating a lot of high-iron foods. It's not unusual for vegetarian women to have lower levels of ferritin even if their hematocrit and hemoglobin are in the normal range.

ALERT

Large doses of iron can be toxic. Only take the amount of iron recommended by your health care provider. Store iron supplements out of the reach of children and make sure that your bottle has a childproof cap if there are children in the house.

Iron-deficiency anemia can lead to pica—craving nonfood items such as ice, clay, dirt, paper, or laundry starch as well as flour or cornstarch. If you experience these types of cravings, let your health care provider know. Nonfood items can contain toxins or contaminants that could be harmful to your baby and can interfere with nutrient absorption.

Supplement Strategy

In order to make sure you're getting enough iron, your health care provider will recommend an iron-enriched prenatal vitamin-mineral supplement, an iron supplement, or both. The level of iron you need will depend on your iron status. For example, the CDC recommends an iron supplement of 30 milligrams per day beginning at your first prenatal visit. If you're diagnosed with iron deficiency, a higher dose supplement, 60–120 milligrams, may be prescribed. Talk to your health care provider to determine how much iron is right for you.

It's best to take iron supplements between meals or with a source of vitamin C (a glass of juice, for instance) to help your body absorb iron. If morning sickness is making it difficult to keep between-meal iron supplements down, temporarily try taking them with a meal.

Some women find that iron supplements, especially higher dose supplements, lead to constipation. This may not affect you; vegan diets are typically quite high in fiber, so constipation is not something many vegans experience. If your iron supplements do seem to be constipating, try a daily glass of prune juice. Not only will this help make things move, it's also a good way to add some iron. Making sure you're eating plenty of high-fiber foods like dried beans, whole grains, fruits, and vegetables can also help with constipation.

If you're taking an iron supplement, don't be concerned if you notice that your stools look darker than usual. This is a common side effect of high doses of iron and is not harmful. Of course, if you see blood in your stools, you should contact your health care provider.

High-dose iron supplements can interfere with the absorption of other minerals. If you're taking a higher dose of iron, your health care provider may check to make sure you're getting enough zinc and copper.

Vegan Zinc Sources

Zinc plays an important role in your baby's development, so it's a mineral to be aware of. Many foods that are good sources of iron are also good sources of zinc. Prenatal supplements also typically contain zinc.

Zinc deficiencies are rare in the United States. Mild zinc deficiencies may lead to poor appetite, a reduced sense of taste, and slower wound healing.

Zinc requirements go up with pregnancy. Coincidentally, the amount of zinc that you absorb from meals increases also. Just as with iron, however, phytates and other substances in foods from plants can interfere with zinc absorption. Similarly to iron, there are strategies that you can use to make the most of food sources of zinc.

An easy meal that provides as much as half of the zinc recommendation for pregnancy consists of ¾ cup of curried chickpeas, 1½ cups of quinoa, and ½ cup of sautéed mushrooms. Add a sprinkling of chopped cashews to supply even more zinc. Key zinc sources in this meal are the chickpeas, quinoa, and mushrooms. Dried beans, whole grains, and zinc-fortified foods are all excellent zinc choices for vegans.

Some breakfast cereals are fortified with zinc, as are some veggie "meats" and energy bars. If you're looking for higher zinc brands, check the Nutrition Facts label at the grocery store. Just as for iron, adding a spoonful or two of wheat germ to hot cereals or other grain dishes adds extra zinc.

Vegetables that have the highest amounts of zinc include mushrooms, spinach, peas, corn, and asparagus. Fruits are not an especially good way to get zinc. Dark chocolate is not just a good way to get iron, it also provides zinc—and has more of either of these minerals than milk chocolate.

The following vegan foods are especially good zinc sources:

1. Zinc-fortified breakfast cereals (up to 15 milligrams of zinc in 1 ounce of cereal)
2. Wheat germ (2.7 milligrams in 2 tablespoons)
3. Zinc-fortified veggie "meats" (up to 1.8 milligrams in 1 ounce)
4. Zinc-fortified energy bars (up to 5.2 milligrams in a bar)
5. Adzuki beans (4 milligrams in 1 cup)
6. Tahini (1.4 milligrams in 2 tablespoons)
7. Chickpeas (2.4 milligrams in 1 cup)
8. Black-eyed peas (2.2 milligrams in 1 cup)
9. Lentils (2.6 milligrams in 1 cup)
10. Peanuts, peanut butter (close to 2 milligrams in 2 tablespoons)

Making the Most of Zinc

While zinc absorption is lower from beans and grains than it is from meats, there are definitely techniques that you can use to raise the amount of zinc you absorb from a vegan diet. Zinc is better absorbed from yeast-raised breads than from quick breads or muffins that are leavened with baking powder or baking soda. That doesn't mean that you can't eat quick breads or muffins; just be aware that yeast-raised breads provide more zinc. Zinc absorption is higher from fermented foods like sauerkraut, soy sauce, and tempeh. If you are into sprouting, you're in luck. Sprouting grains and beans reduces their phytate content and makes it easier to absorb the zinc in these foods.

These ideas are all ways to fine-tune your dietary zinc levels. If you don't have time to bake your own bread or sprout lentils, don't worry. Just check your prenatal supplement to make sure that it supplies zinc and take it regularly.

CHAPTER 5

Vegan Nutrition: Building Bones and Teeth

Calcium and vitamin D are important nutrients for building strong bones and teeth. Both of these nutrients can be supplied by a vegan diet. For example, especially good sources of calcium include leafy greens—think kale and bok choy. Vitamin D is added to foods, and made by your body after you've been in the sun. Many nondairy milks are fortified with both calcium and vitamin D in forms that are easily absorbed. Your body even provides extra help—you absorb more calcium when you're pregnant.

Key Nutrients for Bone Health

Together, calcium and vitamin D are thought of as the most important nutrients for healthy bones, but other vitamins and minerals, along with protein, are also needed for bone health. When bones first develop, protein forms a sort of scaffolding that is filled in with the minerals calcium and phosphorus. Calcium and phosphorus are what make bones hard and unlikely to break. Vitamin D plays an important role because it increases the amount of calcium that is absorbed. Your bones need a constant supply of calcium because they are always changing and rebuilding, even when you're no longer growing. And, of course, when you're pregnant, you need calcium to form your baby's bones.

Other important nutrients for healthy bones include phosphorus, vitamin K, vitamin B_{12}, riboflavin, protein, and vitamin B_6. In other words, eating a well-balanced diet is one of the best things you can do to make sure that your bones get the nutrients they need.

FACT

Besides its important role in building strong bones, calcium is also important for building strong teeth. Even though your baby's teeth won't appear until sometime in the first year after birth, they're developing during pregnancy. Calcium also helps make baby's jawbone strong.

And it's not just nutrition that's important for bones. Exercise, especially weight-bearing exercise, such as walking, running, low-impact or step aerobics, is important throughout your life to make sure that your bones stay strong as you get older. Exercise while pregnant won't really help your baby's bones, but it has other benefits.

Baby's Bone Development

Your baby's skeleton begins to develop in the third week after conception. Twenty-four weeks later, the bones are fully developed. At this point, baby's bones are not hard like mature bones are; they are still soft and bend easily. By the time your baby is born, she'll have accumulated close to an ounce of calcium, most of it in her bones, all supplied by you. Your baby's bones will continue to mature after birth and will become harder and longer with time. Some bones will fuse together as the baby develops, so the total number of bones in adulthood is less than the number at birth.

Calcium Needs

Throughout your pregnancy, you will be meeting your baby's calcium needs. The calcium from foods you eat will move from your intestines, into your blood, through the placenta, and to your baby. Although your baby's bones are growing throughout pregnancy, the last trimester is peak growth time. During that trimester, he'll need 200–250 milligrams of calcium a day—a little less than the amount of calcium in a cup of fortified soymilk (if you absorbed all of that calcium). Since you only absorb a third or less of dietary calcium, the RDA for calcium is higher than 200–250 milligrams.

With pregnancy, calcium needs are higher in order to maintain your bones and to supply calcium for your baby's bone and teeth development. Remarkably, your body compensates for the increased calcium needs by pumping up the amount of calcium that you absorb from your food. Early in pregnancy, the amount of calcium you absorb doubles; higher calcium absorption continues throughout your pregnancy. Since calcium absorption is so high in pregnancy, the recommendation for how much calcium you need doesn't increase above what it was prepregnancy. So if you were getting the amount of calcium that you needed before you were pregnant and you're eating similar foods now, chances are good that you're meeting your calcium needs.

Vegan Calcium Sources

Almost every one of the food groups in a vegan's diet has foods that can markedly add to calcium intake. From nuts and seeds to vegetables, fruits, and fruit juices, foods from all of these groups as well as beans and grains can provide calcium that is very well absorbed. Typically, about 30 percent of the calcium in dairy products is absorbed. That same 30 percent is absorbed from foods fortified with calcium. Green vegetables are the true prize-winners when it comes to calcium; more than half of the calcium in green vegetables like kale, broccoli, and Chinese cabbage is absorbed.

Vegetables Provide Calcium

With a few exceptions, if a vegetable is green and has leaves, it is a good source of calcium. Calcium-rich vegetables include bok choy, broccoli, Chinese cabbage, collard greens, kale, mustard greens, and turnip greens. Even some nonleafy vegetables, including okra and butternut squash, supply some calcium. Calcium is added to some commercial vegetable juices also—check the label for 30 percent calcium.

ALERT

A few foods contain oxalic acid, a substance that can interfere with calcium absorption from those foods. While food charts make spinach, Swiss chard, beet greens, rhubarb, and sweet potatoes look like good sources of calcium, the oxalic acid in these foods keeps you from absorbing much calcium from them.

You could get close to the calcium RDA of 1,000 milligrams by eating about 4–5 cups of cooked kale, collards, or turnip greens, and for someone who really loves greens, that is not impossible. Assuming you'd prefer to rely on some other foods also, it's still possible to get a generous dose of calcium from green vegetables without eating several bowls of them a day. You can add finely chopped greens to soups, chili, or other stews, curries, pasta sauce, grains (green rice, anyone?), and mashed potatoes. Try sautéing chopped greens in a little olive oil and seasoning them with garlic and lemon juice. Add greens to stir-fries. Mild, tender greens like kale can be finely shredded and added to tossed salads or used in place of lettuce on burritos or wraps.

Beans and Soy Foods Supply Calcium, Too

Dried beans are another calcium source for vegans. Soybeans, black beans, great northern beans, and navy beans are especially high in calcium. Other dried beans, while not superstars, can still add to your calcium intake.

Since soybeans are high in calcium, foods made from soybeans also supply calcium. Tempeh, soy nuts (roasted soybeans), TVP, and tofu are all naturally rich calcium sources. Tofu is made by mixing soymilk with a mineral salt to make the soymilk firm up (sort of like making cheese). Many tofu makers use nigari (magnesium chloride) as a coagulating agent. Calcium sulfate is another coagulating agent that is also used. Tofu made with calcium sulfate is especially high in calcium; however, if you can only find tofu made with nigari, you are still getting some calcium from the soybeans that were used to make tofu.

ALERT

If you're relying on calcium-fortified soymilk or other plant milks as one of your calcium mainstays, be sure to shake the milk thoroughly before pouring it. That will help to make sure that the calcium is mixed in and doesn't settle to the bottom of the carton.

If you purchase calcium-fortified soymilk, you'll be buying soymilk that has calcium added to it. This calcium is well absorbed. Many brands of soymilk supply as much calcium per cup as cow's milk. Check the label of your favorite brand to make sure calcium has been added. Some brands of vegan cheese and yogurt are also fortified with calcium.

Don't Forget Nuts, Seeds, Fruits, Grains, and Other Foods

While greens, tofu, and calcium-fortified soymilk can supply enough calcium to meet your needs, there are many other foods that are either naturally high in calcium or that are fortified with calcium.

Almond butter, sesame seeds, and tahini are the best sources of calcium when it comes to nuts and seeds. Fruits are not especially high in calcium with the exception of figs—a cup of dried figs has almost as much calcium as a cup of collard greens. Dried figs can also help with the constipation that can be a feature of late pregnancy. Try eating a few figs for snacks or adding them to hot cereal.

If you look in the supermarket refrigerated or frozen section, you'll see that many brands of juice, especially orange juice, are calcium-fortified. If you're trying to increase your calcium, choosing a fortified juice is an easy way to do it.

Many commercial breakfast cereals are fortified with calcium. The Nutrition Facts label can help you decide which cereals are good calcium sources—look for 30 percent or more of the calcium DV in a serving. Plant milks like rice milk, almond milk, and oat milk are also often fortified with calcium.

Adding a spoonful of blackstrap molasses to hot cereals, muffin batter, baked beans, or stews is another way to boost your calcium intake. A table-spoon of blackstrap molasses provides 200 milligrams of calcium.

While many foods vegans eat supply calcium, the following foods are some of the highest sources:

1. Calcium-fortified plant milks
2. Dried figs
3. Tofu (especially prepared with calcium sulfate)
4. Collard greens
5. Kale
6. Turnip greens and bok choy
7. Calcium-fortified orange juice
8. Blackstrap molasses
9. Soybeans
10. Navy beans

Calcium Supplements

Many prenatal vitamin-mineral supplements do not supply much cal-cium. Check the label of the brand that you are using. Ideally, you would be getting the calcium you need from foods. If your diet is low in calcium, how-ever, and your prenatal has little or no calcium, a separate calcium supple-ment may be needed. The two most common forms of calcium supplements are calcium carbonate and calcium citrate. Each kind has some advantages.

Calcium carbonate is usually less expensive and fewer tablets may be needed. It is absorbed best when taken with food. The drawback of tak-ing calcium supplements with foods is that the calcium interferes with iron absorption.

Calcium supplements made with calcium citrate can be taken between meals, so there's less chance that they'll interfere with iron absorption.

Calcium supplements may cause you to have more gas or to feel bloated or constipated. If that happens, try to take several smaller doses of calcium supplements throughout the day or try a different brand.

Myths and Facts about Calcium

One of the simplest myths about calcium to dispel is the idea that dairy products are needed to get enough calcium. Look around at plant-eating animals like horses, cows, and hippopotamuses—their massive bones are all made from calcium from plant foods. Milk is not a part of their adult diet.

Protein and Calcium

The relationship between protein, calcium, and bone health is a complex one. Older research suggested that people on very high-protein diets had a lot of calcium in their urine. In other words, they were losing calcium rather than storing it. This research led to the idea that people whose diets were lower in protein lost less calcium. Since their calcium losses were lower, the theory was that people on lower protein diets would not need as much calcium. Some vegans seized on this idea and guessed that vegans wouldn't need as much calcium as meat eaters do since the vegan diet is typically lower in protein.

ALERT

Very high intakes of calcium have been associated with kidney stones, not something anyone wants. It's unlikely you'll go over the safe upper limit for calcium of 2,500 milligrams a day from your diet, but if you're also taking calcium supplements, it can happen. Check the labels of all supplements for their calcium content.

More recent studies have found that both adequate protein and adequate calcium are needed to produce strong bones less likely to fracture. Vegans should try to meet the RDA for calcium and to have enough protein in their diets. (For more on protein, see Chapter 3.)

Vitamin D: The Sunshine Vitamin

Vitamin D is known as the sunshine vitamin because your body makes vitamin D when your skin is exposed to the sun. Vitamin D is needed for your body to absorb calcium, so it is often linked to healthy bones. Only a few foods contain vitamin D naturally—mushrooms are one example of a vegan food that provides some vitamin D. Some mushrooms that have recently become available are exposed to ultraviolet light, which increases their vitamin D content. The main dietary source of vitamin D for many Americans is the vitamin D added to cow's milk. Vegan sources of vitamin D are also fortified foods; vitamin D is added to some brands of plant milks, fruit juices, and breakfast cereals.

Vitamin D needs do not increase in pregnancy. The RDA for vitamin D in pregnancy is 600 IU, the same as for nonpregnant women.

Vitamin D Production

It doesn't take much sun exposure to make all the vitamin D that you need. If you're fair skinned and can be out in the summer sun, experts estimate that you need about five to ten minutes a few times a week on your arms and face to meet your needs. This is a very rough estimate, however, and many factors can affect the production of vitamin D.

Sunscreen and clothing block vitamin D production, so if you'd like to get vitamin D from the sun, wait a few minutes before putting on sunscreen or covering up. Remember though, that use of sunscreen is important to lower your risk for skin cancer.

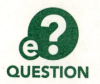

QUESTION

Can I get too much vitamin D from the sun?
Your body only produces the vitamin D that it needs, so even with a large dose of sunlight you won't make excessive amounts of vitamin D. Of course, too much sun has potential to increase your risk of skin cancer, so don't overdo it!

If your skin is darker or if you live where there's a lot of air pollution or it's a cloudy day, you will need more sun exposure to make vitamin D. Winter sun in the northern part of the United States is not strong enough to promote vitamin D production. If you live in the north in the winter, don't get out in the sun that much, or use sunscreen or protective clothing whenever you're outside, you'll need to know about other ways to meet your vitamin D needs.

Vitamin D Sources for Vegans

Look to fortified foods and supplements for most of your vitamin D. Vitamin D is added to many brands of plant milks including almond milk, hemp milk, coconut milk, rice milk, and soymilk. Some brands of dairy look-alikes (like yogurt and cheese) also have vitamin D added. Breakfast cereals, juices, and energy bars are some other products often fortified with vitamin D.

Fresh mushrooms, identified on the label as being a good source of vitamin D, have been exposed to ultraviolet light that stimulated the mushroom's production of vitamin D. A 3-ounce serving of these mushrooms has about 400 IU of vitamin D or about two-thirds of the recommended daily intake.

Vitamin D supplements are another option. Many calcium supplements also contain vitamin D and so do most prenatal supplements. Before taking extra vitamin D (beyond what is in your prenatal), check with your health care provider or RD to make sure you're not overdoing this vitamin.

Vitamin D_2 Versus Vitamin D_3

Vitamin D is found in two different forms in supplements and fortified foods. Vitamin D_2, also called ergocalciferol, is made from yeast exposed to ultraviolet light. Vitamin D_2 is a vegan form of vitamin D. Vitamin D_3, also called cholecalciferol, is made from lanolin from sheep's wool and is not considered vegan. Both forms of vitamin D are effective ways to meet requirements.

Most, although not all, brands of soymilk and other plant milks are fortified with vitamin D_2. Breakfast cereals and orange juice are commonly fortified with vitamin D_3, as is margarine. High vitamin D mushrooms contain vitamin D_2; supplements may contain either variety. If you would prefer to avoid vitamin D_3, check the ingredient listing on products that you use. Most products will identify either vitamin D_3 or vitamin D_2 in the list of ingredients. If a package simply says vitamin D, you can contact the company to ask about the kind of vitamin D added to that product.

CHAPTER 6

Vegan Nutrition: Building a Healthy Nervous System

Some of the most exciting times for a mom are when her baby first makes eye contact, smiles, and begins to talk. It's as if you can see your baby's brain growing as one new skill after another is acquired. Just like all of baby's systems, the nervous system (including the brain and nerves) develops rapidly before birth and in the weeks and months after birth. Vitamin B_{12}, folic acid, iodine, and DHA are all nutrients that, along with protein, are needed to build a healthy nervous system.

Vitamin B$_{12}$ Is Essential for Vegans

Although only a very small amount (less than a gram) of vitamin B$_{12}$ is needed, it is essential for health. Having one or more daily, reliable sources of B$_{12}$ is especially important when you're not only providing for yourself but also responsible for meeting the needs of your unborn, and later (if you're breastfeeding) newborn, baby. Vitamin B$_{12}$ stored in your body may not be available for transportation through the placenta or in breast milk to your baby, but B$_{12}$ from diet or supplements is. That's why it's important to get B$_{12}$ every day from food or supplements.

Vitamin B$_{12}$ plays an important role in developing and maintaining the nervous system. Deficiencies of this nutrient are rare, but when they occur, they can have serious consequences including developmental delays, difficulty walking, and permanent damage to the nervous system.

In nature, all vitamin B$_{12}$ is produced by microorganisms; neither animals nor plants can make B$_{12}$. Vitamin B$_{12}$ is found in meat, milk, eggs, and other animal-based foods because animals eat microorganisms that contain B$_{12}$. There are no reliable plant-based sources of B$_{12}$ other than foods fortified with it. The limited number of nonanimal sources of B$_{12}$ makes it a nutrient vegans have to pay attention to. Getting enough as a vegan is an easy issue to address, but one that is important to be proactive about.

Vegan Sources of Vitamin B$_{12}$

Fortunately for vegans, many food manufacturers add vitamin B$_{12}$ to their products—check labels to see if vitamin B$_{12}$ is added to foods you use. Some vegan products that commonly (or at least sometimes) have vitamin B$_{12}$ added are:

- Plant milks
- Energy bars and protein bars
- Marmite yeast extract
- Tofu
- Vegetarian Support Formula nutritional yeast
- Veggie "meats"
- Breakfast cereals

To learn more about some of these less common foods, see Chapter 9.

Companies have been known to change their product formulation, especially with regard to vitamin fortification. Check the label of foods you rely on for vitamin B_{12} frequently so you're not lulled into thinking a product has vitamin B_{12} when it no longer does.

Nutritional Yeast

Nutritional yeast, a mild-tasting, light yellow flake or powder, is a good source of B_{12} if the yeast is grown with a medium containing B_{12}. Nutritional yeast containing B_{12} is commonly available in packages and in bulk food bins. Check the label to make sure the product you are using contains it. A tablespoon of Vegetarian Support Formula nutritional yeast flakes supplies 4 micrograms of B_{12}.

Nutritional yeast is a versatile ingredient that can be added to many dishes. Here are some ideas:

- Sprinkle on freshly popped popcorn along with a bit of salt or chili powder
- Mix with bread crumbs and use to top a casserole or in breading
- Add to your favorite scrambled tofu recipe (see Chapter 17)
- Use to add flavor to steamed vegetables, grain and pasta dishes, soups, veggie pizza, and other foods commonly topped with Parmesan cheese (see Chapters 18–20 for some ideas)
- Mix in with mashed potatoes
- Mix in with bread dough to add a cheesy taste to breadsticks or other savory breads
- Use to top breakfast toast (along with vegan margarine)
- Make a nutritional yeast-based dip (see Chapter 22 for dip recipes)

Getting Enough Vitamin B_{12}

Most prenatal vitamins contain vitamin B_{12}. If your prenatal supplies at least 45 percent of the DV for vitamin B_{12} and you take it daily in the amount recommended, you should be set. If your prenatal doesn't supply B_{12}, you'll need to seek out other sources—a separate B_{12} supplement providing at least 2.6 micrograms (some vegan dietitians recommend as much as 25–100 micrograms) or three or more servings of B_{12}-fortified foods daily.

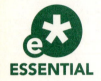

ESSENTIAL

If you're taking vitamin B_{12} in pill form, it should be crushed or chewed before swallowing. This improves the odds that the B_{12} in the pill will be well absorbed. Crushed B_{12} pills can be mixed with applesauce, pudding, or other foods to minimize the taste. Powdered B_{12} in vegan capsules does not need to be chewed.

While people may point out that very few vegans develop B_{12} deficiencies, it's much better to be safe than sorry.

Don't Count on These Foods for Vitamin B_{12}

Foods reported to contain vitamin B_{12} include fermented foods (tempeh, sauerkraut, miso), sea vegetables, shiitake mushrooms, spirulina (algae), and soybeans. None of these foods, in fact no plant foods, contain enough B_{12} to prevent a deficiency. In fact, some of these foods contain a vitamin B_{12} analogue (something that looks like vitamin B_{12} but isn't) that can interfere with B_{12} absorption from other foods.

Folic Acid for Vegans

Folic acid (folate) is another essential vitamin. It's especially important early in pregnancy when the baby's neural tube is being formed. The neural tube develops into the brain and the spinal cord (the central nervous system). Adequate intake of folic acid while the neural tube is formed reduces the risk of birth defects like spina bifida.

A typical vegan diet includes many foods that are good sources of folate, including dried beans, leafy vegetables, oranges, orange juice, and peanuts. Folic acid is in breads, cereals, rice, pasta, flour, and other grain products.

Because folic acid is so important, the CDC recommends that pregnant women take a vitamin or eat a fortified breakfast cereal that contains 100 percent of the DV for folic acid every day. In fact, because a woman may not be aware that she is pregnant at the time when the fetus' neural tube starts to form, the CDC's recommendations for folic acid apply to all women of child-bearing age, not just pregnant women.

DHA's Role

Docosahexaenoic acid (DHA) is a fatty acid most commonly found in the oil from fish. However, vegans can get DHA without having to eat salmon, tuna, or other fish. DHA, categorized as an omega-3 fatty acid, plays a role in the development of your baby's vision. DHA may also affect your baby's cognitive development.

In the last trimester, the fetus stores DHA in her brain and in her retina (a part of the eye). If your diet is low in DHA, stored DHA from your body will be used to meet your fetus' needs. Some experts fear this will make your stores of DHA too low.

There is a great deal of interest in DHA, and many research studies being conducted. Some studies have found that blood levels of DHA in pregnant vegetarians are lower than in pregnant nonvegetarians. Whether or not this makes any difference is not known. Researchers have also found that if the mother has a higher DHA intake in pregnancy, her infant's visual acuity at four months is improved, although this effect is not seen at age six months. Small improvements in developmental function are also seen in infants whose mothers had higher DHA intakes in pregnancy.

DHA Without Fish

When it comes to DHA, vegans can get some DHA indirectly by taking another omega-3 fatty acid called ALA that is converted to DHA. Addition-ally, vegans can get DHA by taking vegan DHA supplements.

Make Your Own DHA

Alpha-linolenic acid (ALA) is another omega-3 fatty acid your body is able to use to make DHA. Rates of production are slow, however, so it is unlikely you can make all the DHA you need in pregnancy. Still, you can get some DHA by making your own.

Besides being a building block for DHA, ALA is important on its own, so even if you're not counting on it to make DHA, having good sources of ALA is a part of a healthy vegan diet. Foods that are especially high in ALA are flaxseeds, flaxseed oil, canola oil, hemp seeds, hemp seed oil, walnut oil, and walnuts.

Flaxseeds are small, dark brown seeds with a slightly nutty taste. You can find them in breakfast cereals, breads, and even snack crackers and tortilla chips. Whole flaxseeds add a nice crunch, but that's about all; the fact is that most of them pass through your body undigested because of their hull. In order to release the ALA from flaxseeds, the seeds need to be ground into flaxseed meal, a powder that can be used in baking or added to smoothies. You can grind your own using a spice or coffee grinder or purchase it already ground. Flaxseed meal should be stored in the refrigerator or freezer.

FACT

Flaxseed oil is added to many foods. If you'd like to get more omega-3 fats, look for peanut butter or vegan margarine with added flaxseed oil. Of course, you can make your own flaxseed oil-enhanced peanut butter by mixing a spoonful of flaxseed oil with a couple of spoonfuls of peanut butter.

Flaxseed oil can be added to foods after they have been cooked, but should not be used for cooking—the heat destroys the healthy fats. It's fine to mix flaxseed oil with steamed vegetables, cooked pasta, hot cereals, or other warm foods. It can be used to make salad dressings and be added to smoothies without altering their taste. Just like flaxseeds, flaxseed oil should be stored in the refrigerator.

Hemp seeds and hemp seed oil come from the hemp plant. You may have noticed hemp seeds, hemp milk, hemp flour, hemp oil, and hemp butter as well as products with added hemp at the grocery store. Shelled hemp seeds can be sprinkled onto foods or used in baking. Hemp seed butter can be used in place of peanut butter, and hemp flour is a gluten-free product.

DHA from Microalgae

Some people think fish are a good source of DHA because fish make their own DHA. Wrong. Fish, like people, don't make DHA. Fish actually get DHA the same way vegans (and other nonfish eaters) do, by eating algae. Certain algaes naturally contain DHA. The oil from these algaes is used to make vegan DHA supplements and to fortify foods with nonfish DHA.

FACT

Besides being a good source of ALA, hemp seeds supply other essential nutrients. Two tablespoons of shelled hemp seeds have about 80 calories and supply as much protein as ½ cup of beans. That same amount of hemp seeds provides generous amounts of iron, folic acid, and zinc.

A workshop sponsored by the National Institutes of Health (NIH) and the International Society for the Study of Fatty Acids and Lipids (ISSFAL) recommended an intake of 300 milligrams daily of DHA for pregnant and lactating women. The easiest way to get DHA is to take a DHA supplement.

If you are interested in finding foods with vegan DHA, check the ingredient listing for DHA algal oil. Not all foods that contain DHA algal oil are vegan; the oil is also added to some brands of cow's milk, yogurt, and other nonvegan products.

Some prenatal supplements contain vegan DHA. Again, check for microalgal oil on the ingredient list. Separate vegan DHA supplements are also available. See the resource list in Appendix A.

Iodine Is Important Also

Iodine, a mineral that you may have heard of because it is added to iodized salt, is essential for the development of your baby's brain. Worldwide, iodine deficiency in pregnancy and early childhood is the single most important preventable cause of brain damage. Iodine needs are higher in pregnancy to be sure your baby gets enough iodine for brain development.

Because of variations in soil iodine in the United States, in 1924, the government approved the addition of iodine to salt. To see if the salt you use is iodized, check the package. Commercial sea salt contains variable amounts of iodine; at least one brand has iodine added. Three-quarters of a teaspoon of iodized salt provides enough iodine to meet the RDA for pregnancy.

Many people don't use this much salt. If you don't or if you use sea salt or other noniodized salt, you may need an iodine supplement. Many prenatal supplements contain iodine, but not all do. The American Thyroid Association recommends that pregnant women take a daily prenatal vitamin that contains 150 micrograms of iodine.

Sea vegetables like nori and kombu can provide some iodine, but amounts are variable. Some sea vegetables are very high in iodine. Arame, hiziki, and kombu are examples of high-iodine sea vegetables, but because excess iodine can cause health problems for you and your baby, you should limit use of these high-iodine sea vegetables during pregnancy.

CHAPTER 7

Vitamins and Supplements

Many vegans' diets are better than typical American diets. Fruits, vegetables, whole grains, nuts, and dried beans that are mainstays of vegan diets supply key vitamins and minerals. Still, women's diets are often low in nutrients such as iron, zinc, magnesium, and vitamins E and D. Pregnancy is a great opportunity to evaluate and revise your dietary habits, if necessary. Morning sickness, lack of time, and other situations can sabotage your best intentions; prenatal and other dietary supplements can help ensure you're getting the nutrients you need.

Vitamins and Minerals in Pregnancy

In pregnancy, and later when breastfeeding, women need more calories, protein, and some vitamins and minerals to meet the needs of their growing baby. Most of these nutrients can come from your regular diet, but supplements may be needed for some nutrients that are commonly in short supply. The following chart shows how recommendations for some vitamins and minerals change in pregnancy and during breastfeeding.

RECOMMENDED DIETARY ALLOWANCE FOR VEGAN WOMEN AGE 19 AND OLDER			
Nutrient	Nonpregnant	Pregnant	Breastfeeding
Calcium	1000mg	1000mg	1000mg
Iodine	150mcg	220mcg	290mcg
Magnesium	310–320mg	350–360mg	310–320mg
Iron	32mg	49mg	16mg
Zinc	8mg	11mg	12mg
Vitamin A	700mcg	770mcg	1300mcg
Vitamin D	15mcg	15mcg	15mcg
Vitamin E	15mg	15mg	19mg
Vitamin K	90mcg	90mcg	90mcg
Thiamin	1.1mg	1.4mg	1.4mg
Riboflavin	1.1mg	1.4mg	1.6mg
Niacin	14mg	18mg	17mg
Vitamin B_6	1.3mg	1.9mg	2.0mg
Folate	400mcg	600mcg	500mcg
Vitamin B_{12}	2.4mcg	2.6mcg	2.8mcg
Vitamin C	75mg	85mg	120mg

RDAs from the Food and Nutrition Board, Institute of Medicine

Although recommendations are higher in pregnancy for magnesium, vitamin A, thiamin, riboflavin, niacin, vitamin B_6, and vitamin C, it's likely that as you increase the amount of food you eat you'll also get more of these nutrients (assuming you're eating a reasonably healthy diet). The RDA for iron in pregnancy is challenging for most women to meet from diet alone. Zinc can also be difficult, especially if you're relying mainly on beans and grains as zinc sources. Folate and iodine supplements are recommended in pregnancy. Vegan women need to use either fortified foods or a supplement to meet vitamin B_{12} needs.

Women who are pregnant should not take regular vitamins; they could be too low in some nutrients and too high in others. Ask your health care provider about special prenatal supplements, which contain the vitamins and minerals you will need during your pregnancy. Be sure to tell your health care provider about any vitamins you are already taking before adding a prenatal vitamin supplement.

Choosing a Prenatal Vitamin/Mineral Supplement

Your health care provider may recommend a specific brand of prenatal vitamins because she likes the amounts and kinds of vitamins and minerals in it. You may opt to use this recommendation, but it may or may not be vegan. If taking a vegan prenatal supplement is important to you, discuss options with your health care provider. You can research brands and nutrients supplied by each product online and compare available vegan supplements to the supplement your provider recommends.

A good place to start researching what is available is on websites of companies that make vegan supplements. These include VegLife (*www.veglife .com*), DEVA (*www.devanutrition.com*), Freeda (*www.freedavitamins.com*), Country Life (*www.country-life.com*), and Rainbow Light (*www.rainbowlight .com*). Websites of companies carrying vegan products can also be helpful. See Appendix A for some ideas.

If you are choosing a vegan prenatal supplement, you will need to be sure it meets your needs for essential nutrients low in your diet. A visit to an RD is one way to assess your diet; another way is to look ahead to Chapter 8's food guide to see if your diet generally meets recommendations. Expert groups suggest that pregnant women take a 400mcg folic acid supplement as well as 150mcg of iodine. Having a prenatal supplement that provides these nutrients reduces the number of pills you have to swallow. Other nutrients that can be challenging for vegans in pregnancy include iron, zinc, vitamin B_{12}, calcium, and vitamin D. If your diet doesn't meet your needs for these nutrients, look for a vegan prenatal supplement that can provide at least some of the amount needed and plan to get the rest from your food.

Share what you've learned with your provider and get his approval of any supplement you want to use. Be aware that prenatal supplements vary in terms of which nutrients and the amount of each nutrient that is included. For example, several brands of vegan prenatal supplements do not supply iodine and the amount of zinc ranges from two-thirds to three times the zinc recommendation.

If you have questions about a specific supplement, including whether or not it is vegan, contact the manufacturer for more information.

Supplement Quality

Some independent organizations assess the quality of certain dietary supplements. They check to be sure the supplement contains what it says it does on the label. These quality certifications do not mean the product is safe or effective; the organizations only assess the manufacturing process. Supplement manufacturers are not required to participate in this type of evaluation program. Organizations that evaluate supplements include:

- Consumer Lab (*www.consumerlab.com*)
- NSF International (*www.nsf.org*)
- U.S. Pharmacopeia (*www.usp.org*)
- Natural Products Association TruLabel program (*www.npainfo.org*)

Questions about the manufacturing process or possible contaminants can also be directed to supplement manufacturers.

Iron Supplements

Iron needs are high in pregnancy to support your increased blood volume and to stock iron stores for your baby. Add on the higher iron recommendations for vegetarians and it's virtually impossible to meet iron needs from diet alone, even with careful planning. See Chapter 4 for more information about iron.

Most pregnant women take some sort of iron supplement, either in their prenatal supplement or separately. Your provider will check your blood to assess your iron status. This information will help him determine how much supplemental iron you need to take.

ALERT

If your health care provider recommends you take supplemental iron, be sure to tell her about any medications you are using. Some drugs should not be taken with iron supplements.

Most prenatal supplements contain either 18 milligrams or 27 milligrams of iron. This, in conjunction with good dietary sources of iron, may be enough or your provider may want you to take an additional low-dose iron supplement. If you're diagnosed with iron deficiency, a higher dose supplement, 60–120 milligrams of iron, may be prescribed. Talk to your health care provider to determine how much iron is right for you.

Additional Supplements

In addition to a standard prenatal supplement and possibly iron, you may be wondering about additional supplements. Here is what several expert groups suggest. The CDC recommends that pregnant women get 400 micrograms daily of folic acid from supplements or fortified foods. The American Thyroid Association recommends that pregnant women take a prenatal vitamin that contains 150 micrograms of iodine every day. A workshop sponsored by several scientific groups recommended a DHA intake of 300 milligrams daily in pregnancy. The RDA for vitamin B_{12} for pregnancy is 2.6 micrograms, which can come from supplements or fortified foods. If these nutrients in these amounts are not being supplied by your prenatal supplement (or by fortified foods, if that is an option), let your doctor know so that other sources can be explored.

If you need to take high-dose iron supplements, your health care provider may recommend a supplement of zinc and copper as well. Large amounts of iron can interfere with zinc and copper absorption.

Supplement Timing

Some supplements are better absorbed if they are taken with meals; some are better taken between meals. It's most important that you do take any necessary supplements, and figuring out the best timing improves the odds that you'll get the maximum benefit from the supplement.

Take iron supplements between meals to promote better absorption. Iron absorption can also be enhanced by taking your supplement with a vitamin C source such as orange juice or fresh tangerine juice. Remember that tea and coffee contain substances that can inhibit your absorption of iron (as well as calcium), so try to avoid using these to wash down supplements.

If you're suffering from morning sickness and find it difficult to keep your supplements down, you should try taking them with a meal. As your morning sickness improves, you can return to the between-meals dosing schedule.

If you are taking a calcium supplement, it should be taken separately from your iron supplement or from a prenatal supplement that contains iron. Calcium carbonate supplements are best absorbed with food.

The timing of other supplements—vitamin B_{12}, folic acid, DHA, iodine— is not that important. What is important is to regularly use any supplements recommended by your health care provider.

Too Much of a Good Thing—Avoiding Vitamin Excess

Vitamin and mineral supplements may seem like harmless pills. They are available without a prescription and may be something you take without much thought. In reality, taking too much of some vitamins and minerals can cause health problems. In pregnancy, excesses of some vitamins could be harmful to your baby. For example, very high levels of vitamin A have been linked to birth defects. The simplest way to avoid a problem is to only take the vitamins and minerals that have been approved by your doctor. Dietary supplements are meant to supplement your diet; they do not take the place of eating a healthy, varied vegan diet.

Herbal Supplements in Pregnancy

It's tempting to think that herbal and botanical supplements and remedies are universally safe to use in pregnancy. In reality, just because something seems to come from nature, does not automatically guarantee safety. Think of poison ivy, mistletoe, and some mushrooms—all natural and all potentially dangerous. Even herbs that can be used when you're not pregnant can be harmful to your developing baby. Always check with your provider before taking any sort of supplement or remedy.

Some herbal remedies claim they will help with pregnancy. These claims may or may not be true or based on actual research. Herbal remedies and "natural products" do not have to be approved by the FDA for safety or truth in labeling. Makers of herbal remedies do not have to determine whether or not their products are safe to use in pregnancy, either.

The National Center for Complementary and Alternative Medicine (NCCAM) provides guidance on the use of some herbs in pregnancy. A partial list of products to avoid in pregnancy includes:

- Products that contain bitter orange, black cohosh, and red clover should not be used due to a lack of safety evidence. These should also be avoided by nursing women.
- Ephedra, yohimbe, and goldenseal should be avoided in pregnancy and when breastfeeding.
- Cat's claw should be avoided because of its use in the past to prevent pregnancy.
- Chasteberry can affect hormone levels.
- Fenugreek, feverfew, and licorice can induce premature delivery.

This is not an all-inclusive list of products to avoid. Before using any herbal or botanical product, consult your health care provider. In addition to affecting your baby's health, these products can also interfere with medications and have an effect on conditions like gestational diabetes and high blood pressure.

CHAPTER 8

Vegan Nutrition: Putting It All Together

You've heard it before—whole grains, beans, fruits, vegetables, and nuts are the basis for a healthy vegan diet. But maybe that's not enough. How many servings of vegetables should you be eating now that you're pregnant? Are there foods that you should avoid? A simple vegan food guide for pregnancy can help. And if you'd like even more support, a session with a knowledgeable RD is a very worthwhile undertaking.

Vegan Food Guide for Pregnancy

Many food guides don't work for vegans. Food guides often include a meat group and a dairy group. Even if you replace meat with vegetable protein sources, you're still left with a food group that recommends eating cheese and drinking cow's milk.

This vegan food guide for pregnancy is based on five food groups. All servings listed are the minimum number of servings from each food group. If you are not gaining weight at the recommended rate, you'll need to eat a larger number of servings from the food groups. Be sure to choose a variety of foods from each food group.

RECOMMENDED DAILY FOOD CHOICES FOR VEGAN PREGNANCY	
Food Group	Daily Servings
Grains	6
Dried Beans, Nuts, Milks, and Other Protein-Rich Foods	7
Vegetables	4
Fruits	2
Fats	2

In addition to making food choices based on this food guide, you should also be taking a prenatal supplement that supplies vitamins and minerals including iron, zinc, iodine, vitamin B_{12}, and vitamin D. Supplemental DHA is also recommended in pregnancy. See Chapter 7 for more information on supplements.

Grain Group

The grain group includes breads, tortillas, crackers, bagels, rolls, pastas, rices, cereals, quinoa, and other foods made from grains. Choose whole grains often. A serving from this group is a slice of bread; a tortilla or roll; ½ cup of cooked cereal, grain, or pasta; or 1 ounce of ready-to-eat cereal. This food group provides carbohydrates, calories, fiber, B vitamins, iron, and some protein. Fortified cereals can supply other vitamins and minerals.

Dried Beans, Nuts, Milks, and Other Protein-Rich Foods Group

This food group includes a variety of foods that are good sources of protein for vegans. Many foods in this group also supply iron and zinc and some foods are fortified with calcium, vitamin D, and vitamin B_{12}. A serving from this group is ½ cup of cooked dried beans or peas; ½ cup of tofu, TVP, or tempeh; 1 ounce of veggie "meat"; 2 tablespoons of nut or seed butters; ¼ cup of nuts or soy nuts; or 1 cup of fortified soymilk.

ALERT

The Vegan Food Guide for Pregnancy can also be used when you are breastfeeding. For most food groups, eat the same amounts as you did when you were pregnant. Choose one more serving of protein-rich foods, continue to use prenatal vitamins, and add foods as needed to prevent excess weight loss.

Vegetable Group

This food group includes all vegetables, from avocado to zucchini. Vegetables can be eaten raw or cooked. A serving from this group is ½ cup of cooked vegetables or 1 cup of raw vegetables. Be sure to include some nutrient-rich dark-green vegetables and deep-orange vegetables often. This food group is an especially good source of fiber and vitamins A and C; it supplies some iron and zinc.

Fruit Group

Fruits are especially good sources of vitamins C and A; they also provide fiber and B vitamins. The fruit group includes fresh, frozen, canned, and dried fruits and fruit juices. A serving from this group is a piece of medium fruit; ½ cup of cut up or canned fruit; ¼ cup of dried fruit; or ½ cup of fruit juice.

Fats Group

This group provides calories, vitamin E, and essential fatty acids. Foods in this group include oils, vegan salad dressings and mayonnaise, margarine, and vegan cream cheese. A serving of any of these foods is 1 teaspoon.

Meeting Calcium Needs with the Vegan Food Guide

Vegans get calcium from different food groups rather than only one food group—dairy—as nonvegans do. Green leafy vegetables, fortified soymilk, and almonds are examples of some vegan calcium sources. The table below lists amounts of vegan foods that provide approximately 150 milligrams of calcium. By choosing at least six servings (6 × 150 = 900 mg) from this list and getting the rest of the calcium you need from other foods, you can meet the RDA of 1,000 milligrams of calcium. If you are taking a supplement that contains calcium, you will need fewer servings of calcium-rich foods.

FOODS SUPPLYING APPROXIMATELY 150 MG OF CALCIUM	
Food	Serving Size
Cooked collards or turnip greens	½ cup
Cooked kale or broccoli raab	¾ cup
Cooked bok choy, okra, or mustard greens	1 cup
Cooked broccoli	1½ cups
Calcium-fortified juice (orange or vegetable) or milk (soy, almond, etc)	4 ounces
Calcium-fortified vegan yogurt	3 ounces
Calcium-fortified vegan cheese	¾ ounce
Tofu	2 ounces
Tempeh	¾ cup
Almonds	6 tablespoons
Almond butter or tahini	2 tablespoons
Cooked dried beans	1½ cups (1 cup soybeans)
Dried figs	10
English muffin made with calcium propionate	1½
Blackstrap molasses	2 teaspoons
Calcium-fortified energy bar	½

Meeting the Needs of Multiples

If you're carrying twins, triplets, or other multiples, you'll need more servings from all the food groups; your needs for calories and protein are higher. Protein needs for mothers of twins can be met by adding at least three servings of grains, two servings of protein-rich foods, and one serving of vegetables to the Vegan Food Guide.

Menu Planning

Many women choose to eat three meals and several snacks during pregnancy to stave off hunger pangs and to keep from feeling uncomfortably full as the baby gets bigger. Remember, snacks don't have to be a big production. A piece of fruit and some nuts or trail mix can be a satisfying snack.

Here's a sample menu based on the Vegan Food Guide:

BREAKFAST
- ½ cup oatmeal (1 serving grains)
- 2 tablespoons almond butter (1 serving protein; calcium source)
- 4 ounces calcium-fortified orange juice (1 serving fruit; calcium source)

MIDMORNING SNACK
- ½ bagel (1 serving grains)
- ½ cup hummus (1 serving protein; calcium source)

LUNCH
- Sandwich with 1 slice whole-wheat bread (1 serving grains), 1 ounce vegan deli slices (1 serving protein), and 1 teaspoon vegan mayonnaise (1 serving fats)
- 1 cup mixed greens (1 serving vegetables)
- Medium apple (1 serving fruit)

MIDAFTERNOON SNACK
- ¼ cup cashews (1 serving protein)
- 1 cup baby carrots (1 serving vegetables)

DINNER
- 1 cup pasta with tomato sauce (2 servings grains)
- ½ cup chickpeas (1 serving protein)
- 1 cup collards (2 servings vegetables; calcium source) with 1 teaspoon olive oil (1 serving fats)

BEDTIME SNACK
- 1 ounce ready-to-eat cereal (1 serving grains)
- 8 ounces calcium-fortified soymilk (2 servings protein; calcium source)

You'll probably need to add some more foods in order to support weight gain. This sample menu shows how to meet the minimum number of servings for the Vegan Food Guide. Be sure to choose a variety of foods and use a daily prenatal supplement.

Making Sure You're Doing This Right

Maybe you'd like a bit of help with meal planning or maybe you've been diagnosed with gestational diabetes. These are just some examples of scenarios when a visit to an RD could be helpful. Trying to find an RD? Ask your health care provider for a referral or call your local hospital—most hospitals have RDs who provide outpatient counseling.

Here are some situations where a consultation with an RD could be helpful:

- You have a number of food allergies or intolerances
- You're managing a medical condition and you're vegan and you're pregnant
- You've been diagnosed with gestational diabetes or preeclampsia

- You're carrying twins or other multiples
- You have a history of disordered eating
- You were markedly overweight or underweight before pregnancy
- Your health care provider thinks you are not gaining enough or gaining too much weight
- You or someone close to you is concerned about the adequacy of your diet
- You have significant nausea and vomiting that limits the amount and type of food you can eat
- You've just become vegan, either shortly before or during your pregnancy

Of course, you can also consult an RD for help with menu planning, vegan cooking, shopping, or myriad other issues.

The Best Foods

Eating a variety of foods is always good advice. That way, if one food that you eat is high in vitamin X but low in mineral Y, you're likely to choose another food that will be low in vitamin X but high in mineral Y. Eating a variety of foods lets you relax and not have to worry about keeping track of every nutrient.

Certain foods in each food group are especially good sources of a variety of nutrients. For example, in the grains group, whole grains supply more fiber and more of some vitamins and minerals than their refined counterparts. In the vegetables group, dark-green vegetables and deep-orange vegetables are your best choice. That doesn't mean iceberg lettuce and mushrooms are off limits, just that these less nutrient-rich foods should be balanced with some carrots and kale.

Fresh fruits provide more fiber than more processed fruits or juices. If you choose to use canned fruits, select fruits packed in fruit juice rather than in heavy syrup. Dried beans, tofu, tempeh, soymilk, nuts, and nut butters are excellent choices from the protein-rich foods group. More processed foods like veggie "meats" are often higher in sodium, lower in fiber, and more expensive.

Foods to Limit

Everything in moderation is a standard piece of nutrition advice. While moderation is a reasonable approach to eating, be sure that you know what "moderation" means. Moderation means that after you have eaten the appropriate amounts of nutrient-rich foods, it's all right to have a small (emphasis on small) amount of what are often called junk foods.

Junk foods are foods that you would be just fine, nutritionally speaking, if you never ate them again. The sole nutritional value of these foods is that they provide calories; they're not great sources of protein, vitamins, minerals, or other things you need.

Examples of junk foods are soft drinks, candy, cookies, cake, chips, and greasy snack foods. Remember, just because a food is vegan doesn't mean it's healthy. What's wrong with these foods?

Think of your eating plan like your household budget—you have to make choices to stay on your budget. If you need a certain amount of calories to support weight gain in pregnancy, you don't want to "spend" those calories on non-nutritious foods. Rather, you want to get the best nutrition possible within your allotted calories. If you overdo junk foods, they can displace healthier foods in your diet—not good for you or your baby.

That said, if gaining enough weight is a struggle, judicious use of junk foods can help. Once you've eaten your day's share of healthy foods, you can add calories with some higher calorie, lower nutrient foods.

Finding the Time to Eat Right

Whether you're working a hectic job or home with young children or both, eating right can be a matter of planning ahead. If you're crunched for time, it may seem simpler to just skip a meal or grab something (anything) on the way out the door. Of course, there will be times when that's your only choice. Overall, however, setting up a plan can help you eat well.

Quick and Easy Meals

Having a collection of quick and easy meals in your repertoire can help when your plans to get home early and cook dinner aren't possible. Think of meals that you can make without a cookbook or special ingredients. Keep a stock of different breads and rolls in the freezer. A quick meal can always be some hummus or other spread in a wrap with vegetables and a piece of fruit. Scrambled tofu is a quick meal to put together, especially if you have frozen or fresh vegetables that you can scramble along with the tofu. Look for quick-cooking pasta and either keep jarred or homemade sauce on hand. Keep a stock of veggie burgers and buns in the freezer. With canned vegetarian baked beans and some baby carrots, this is a super-quick meal.

Some families use part of a weekend day to make several meals for the week or to do the prep for meals—chop vegetables, cook potatoes for potato salad later, bake bread or desserts. Make-ahead dishes like casseroles, soups, and stews can be refrigerated and then reheated on nights when there's not a lot of time to cook. Leftovers can be frozen and used in a few weeks to add variety. Be sure to keep a list of what's in your freezer so that you don't find mysterious ice-encrusted packages months later and wonder what they are.

Convenience Foods That Work for You

Foods labeled as "convenience foods" may make you think of junk foods that you dash into a convenience food store and eat as you drive. Actually, convenience foods are any foods that can make it easier for you to get a meal together quickly. Choosing good convenience foods and keeping them on hand is one way to ensure that your nutritional needs are met. Canned beans are an example of a useful convenience food that comes in many varieties. Give them a quick rinse to remove some of the canning brine's salt and then use them in any dish calling for cooked beans.

Precut or frozen vegetables can make it easier to serve vegetables. Look for bags of shredded cabbage or peeled winter squash if time is tight. Keeping frozen fruit on hand means it's easy to make smoothies, fruit crisps, or add fruit to muffins or pancakes.

Smart Snacking

Snacking is a key to getting the foods you need. Early in pregnancy, snacks can help with your fickle appetite and with the need to keep nausea at bay by having food in your stomach. As your pregnancy progresses, you'll be less likely to have room for three large meals a day. Instead, you may choose to eat six or more small meals (a.k.a. snacks) daily.

Some snack ideas include:

- Fresh fruit or a fruit smoothie
- Vegetables with a tofu or bean dip
- Rice cakes or bagel slices with nut butter
- Cereal and soymilk
- Bran or blueberry muffin
- Trail mix
- Energy bar and fruit juice

All of these snack ideas involve minimal preparation time. Dips and muffins can be purchased or prepared on a day when you have time, then kept refrigerated or frozen to use as needed.

Vegan in a Nonvegan Family

Suppose that you are vegan but the rest of your household is not. You could microwave a veggie burger every night, but that's really not a solution. Your partner may want to try some vegan foods or even make some vegan meals for you. You need ideas for vegan foods that everyone will eat.

One approach that many vegans in this situation use is to make meatless dishes that you eat as entrées and that your partner can use as side dishes if he wants to. The recipe section of this book has many ideas that will work well as entrées or side dishes.

Another idea is to make dishes you can eat as is and that your partner can add meat or cheese to. For example, stir-fried vegetables can be supplemented with sautéed tofu or chicken. Cheese or cooked ground beef can be added to pasta sauce or chili.

If you make burritos or tacos, your portion can be filled with beans and veggies and your partner's with meat or cheese. Similarly, baked potatoes can be topped with a bean-based or meat-based sauce.

CHAPTER 9

Vegan Shopping and Ingredients

Soymilk in the dairy case, tofu in the produce cooler, non-dairy frozen desserts next to the ice cream—these days many supermarkets are carrying vegan foods. Depending on your location and your food preferences, you may be able to do all of your food shopping in your neighborhood store. Vegans also choose to shop at food co-ops and natural foods stores that may carry a greater variety of vegan specialty products. And if you'd prefer to grocery shop from home, there are a number of online vegan stores.

Finding Vegan Foods in a Supermarket

Your local supermarket carries an impressive number of vegan-friendly foods. While it may take some time to read labels at first, you'll quickly learn which foods and brands will work for you. You may find that most of your purchases are coming from several sections of the store—produce, canned and dried beans, and the natural foods aisle, perhaps. All of these sections will be places you'll find vegan foods, but if you're willing to explore, you'll find that most areas of the store have some vegan items.

Produce Section

It seems obvious that you'd be a regular in the fresh fruit and vegetable aisle. Besides being the place to find produce, many stores locate vegan and vegetarian items in this section. Look around, you may find tofu, mock meats, dairy alternatives, and vegan salad dressings in this section. Be daring—challenge yourself to try a new fruit or vegetable every week or two. And get to know the produce manager; she can often help you decide if a fruit is ripe or provide ideas for using celeriac or other less common vegetables or fruits.

Deli Section

In many stores, the deli section is where you can find a variety of kinds of hummus as well as olives and pickles. Most brands of hummus are vegan, although it never hurts to check the ingredients list. Some stores have packages of vegan deli "meats" in this section. Prepared salads like coleslaw or potato salad are often made with egg-based mayonnaise, but don't be afraid to ask about vegan items—you may find a roasted potato salad with a vinaigrette dressing or a vegan shredded-vegetable salad. Besides, by asking, you are making the store employees aware that people are looking for vegan options.

Bakery

Finding vegan bread in a supermarket can be challenging. Many breads contain whey (milk derivative), eggs, or honey. Rye breads often appear to be vegan and some traditional French or Italian breads are vegan as well. You may have better luck at a store with a natural foods or ethnic section.

Grocery Section

The grocery section is one part of the store where you can find items you never realized were vegan. It's worthwhile to occasionally spend an hour or so in this section, reading labels and making notes of unexpected "finds." Here are some tips for approaching this section of the store:

- If you're looking for a cracker, steer clear of those with cheese or butter in the product's name. Crackers with whole-wheat flour as the first ingredient are a better choice than those with wheat flour listed first.
- Many canned fruits, beans, and vegetables are vegan. Check vegetable labels for added salt pork, bacon, or other meat ingredients. These are especially common in canned greens and beans.
- Hot cereals like oatmeal, grits, and polenta are often vegan. Often the plain (or original) version will simply have the grain as its ingredient. Check the labels on hot cereals for milk or cheese.
- Many brands of pasta are vegan. Some will have eggs added, especially noodles or fettuccine, so check the label. Pasta sauces may have meat or cheese added; marinara sauces are often vegan.
- The ethnic section of the grocery store can have some interesting items. Look for falafel mix in the Middle Eastern section, lard-free refried beans in the Hispanic section, and unusual dried noodles in the Asian section.
- Some supermarkets also have a natural foods section. Of course, all items are not vegan, but this may be where you will find aseptically packaged soymilk, vegan canned soups, and vegan breakfast cereals.
- While not the healthiest part of the store, the snacks aisle does include vegan potato chips, pretzels, tortilla chips, and other munchables. Watch for added cheese or other dairy products.

Frozen Foods

The frozen foods section is where you'll find frozen vegetables (great for times when the produce drawer is empty and your dinner needs a vegetable), frozen fruits (think smoothies), frozen juice concentrate, and frequently frozen veggie burgers. There may be other surprises like vegan pierogies, vegan soups, and vegan frozen desserts.

Dairy Section

Although you might not expect the dairy aisle to have vegan selections, this is where many supermarkets stock refrigerated soymilk and other plant milks. You may also find fruit juices in this section. In some well-stocked supermarkets, you'll also find nondairy yogurt and margarine.

QUESTION

Are frozen vegetables more nutritious than fresh?
It depends. Frozen vegetables are frequently processed immediately after they're picked to minimize nutrient loss. After harvesting, vegetables lose vitamins with exposure to air and sunlight. So if the fresh broccoli is several days away from when it was picked, it may be significantly lower in some vitamins than frozen broccoli.

If you have favorite vegan products that you've seen in other stores or heard about in magazines or online, ask the manager of your supermarket if it would be possible to stock these. If it's a product you know you like and will use, the manager may be able to order a case for you.

Label Reading

What if you could quickly glance at a food's label and know immediately whether or not it was vegan? Such a simple scheme doesn't really exist today, at least not in any consistent way. The U.S. government does not regulate or require the word "vegan" on food labels. If you see a product labeled "vegan" or some sort of an identification mark, it's probably because either the food company or a nonprofit organization has decided that this product meets their standards. It's more likely you'll need to take a look at the ingredient listing to see if a product meets your criteria to be included in your grocery cart.

FACT

If an ingredient listing contains the term "natural flavors," the USDA's Food Safety and Inspection Service (FSIS) requires that, if the natural flavors are derived from animal sources, the label indicates this. The term "natural flavors" on a label without additional qualification means spices, spice extracts, or essential oils were used to flavor the food.

Some obvious signs that a food isn't vegan are meat, fish, poultry, egg, or dairy ingredients. Then there are ingredients like gelatin, beef broth, lard, and Worcestershire sauce (contains anchovies) that are derived from meat or fish. Dairy-derived ingredients include casein (milk protein), whey, and lactase (milk sugar). Some ingredients sound like they might be dairy derived but aren't, like cocoa butter, cream of tartar, and lactic acid. If this is something you're interested in learning more about, check the resource list in Appendix A.

If you have questions about an ingredient and whether or not it is vegan, contact the food company. They may not be able to tell you, but if they hear the question enough, they'll start checking with their ingredient suppliers and may even try to use nonanimal ingredients.

Natural Food Stores, Food Co-Ops, the Internet, and More

If you have a natural foods store or a food co-op nearby, chances are good that you'll find many vegan products on the shelves and in the bulk food bins. Look for all different kinds of dried beans and grains as well as a variety of vegan mock meats and dairy alternatives. Of course, not all foods in these stores are vegan, so label reading is in order. Some seemingly natural products are animal or insect derived. Did you know that the red color of some juices and candies comes from the dried bodies of female insects? If you'd like to avoid this, don't buy products with carmine or cochineal as an ingredient.

Natural foods stores and food co-ops often have bulk food bins. These are a great way to try a small amount of a new food or spice. If you have allergies, however, beware—cross contamination from one bulk bin to another is highly likely.

FACT

The FDA requires that food labels clearly identify all ingredients derived from the most common food allergens: milk, eggs, fish, shellfish, tree nuts, peanuts, wheat, and soybeans. A product that does not list any of these is not necessarily vegan since it could contain meat.

Just like supermarkets, natural foods stores and food co-ops are often happy to special order items for you. If you don't see what you want, talk to a manager.

Vegans living in areas of the country with limited shopping options as well as vegans who like to support vegan-owned companies often look to web-based businesses. Several companies only sell products that they identify as vegan—everything from vegan chocolate to vegan skin care products and cosmetics. Even refrigerated and frozen items can be shipped.

Prices for products ordered online are often similar to those in stores, but you do have the addition of shipping costs. To save, look for special promotions or combine your order with a friend's to get a volume discount. Appendix A includes examples of some online shopping resources.

Stores catering to ethnic populations can yield exciting foods for vegans. Asian grocery stores often carry mock meats, sauces, noodles, rice, exotic vegetables, and other delights. Kosher food stores often carry dairy substitutes. Stores carrying Asian Indian products may have more varieties of dried beans and rice than you have ever seen, along with fragrant spices.

People who follow the Seventh-Day Adventist religion are encouraged to eat a vegetarian diet. Adventists, as they are called, have a long history of developing creative vegetarian foods, especially mock meats. Adventist stores carry several brands of canned and frozen products, many of which are vegan. If you're wishing for vegan scallops, ham, or chops, you will probably find these soy- or wheat-based products in an Adventist store.

Wherever you live, you can find a generous supply of vegan foods. Although specialty stores can add variety, even in small-town USA, you can buy the grains, beans, fruits, and vegetables that are vegan staples.

Shopping on a Budget

Being vegan can result in a drop in your weekly grocery bill, especially if you're choosing beans and whole grains to replace steaks and lobster. If you are buying a lot of vegan specialty or convenience foods, you may see an increase in your food costs. However, it doesn't have to cost more to be a vegan.

Plan Ahead

While convenience foods and take-out can be lifesavers on nights you just can't face the stove, a steady diet of these foods can drive up food costs. Planning ahead doesn't necessarily mean having detailed menus for every meal (although you can do this), but it does mean having some quickly prepared foods in your cupboard or refrigerator. Inexpensive foods to keep on hand for quick meals include tofu, canned beans, and pasta. Taking a few minutes before your regular grocery store trip to check that you have staple foods on the shelf or on your list can save you from multiple trips to the store—costly in terms of time and money if you tend to impulse shop.

Cook It Yourself

Planning ahead also makes it more likely you'll be able to cook more of your own food. That way you can save for a splurge night out at a favorite restaurant rather than eating less-than-tasty take-out just because it's convenient. Maybe it makes sense to do most of your cooking on days when you and your partner are home. Perhaps you can make several dinners and put them in the freezer or refrigerator for later in the week.

Cooking a large pot of beans and one of grains on the weekend can give you the basics for several meals—stir-fry some vegetables one night, toss in some beans and serve over the grain; another night, combine beans, grains, and a vegan salad dressing for a quick entrée salad. If you like to experiment, try making your own seitan or baking your own bread. Along with cost savings, you'll also have learned a new skill.

Shop Smart

Many vegan staples aren't that expensive. Foods like dried beans and grains are relatively low cost. Specialty foods including plant milks, mock meats, nut butters, and frozen convenience foods can take a chunk out of your food budget. If these foods are important to you, there are some ways to cut costs. Store brands of some specialty foods are available, cost less, and are often of comparable quality compared to name brands. For example, many stores sell their own brand of soymilk at a significantly lower price. Many stores, especially smaller stores or food co-ops, offer a case discount of 10 percent or so. If it's a food you'll be able to use before the expiration date, talk to the manager about purchasing a case or more. When products you use are on sale, stock up. If you have space to store them, you can get six months' worth of your favorite brand of chickpeas or vegan canned soup when it's on sale.

Vegan Ingredients

While specialty items are not an essential part of a vegan diet, some of these foods can add variety or even serve as an easy source of some nutrients. Tofu and soymilk may once have seemed exotic, but now they're showing up in many mainstream supermarkets. Other, less familiar, foods that you may see in recipes and wonder about include seitan (pronounced say-tan), agave, and flaxseeds.

Soy Products

All soy products are made from soybeans. Soybeans are a high-protein bean native to East Asia. They are sold in fresh, frozen, canned, and dried forms. Edamame soybeans are a special variety and are sweeter than traditional soybeans. They look a bit like lima beans and are found in the frozen foods section. Fresh edamame soybeans are sometimes found at farmers' markets and in the produce section. Soybeans should not be eaten raw; cooking makes them more digestible.

Soymilk is made by soaking, grinding, and straining soybeans. It is available in both shelf-stable and refrigerated forms and comes in flavors like vanilla, chocolate, and carob. In mid-December, you can often find eggnog flavored soymilk. Vegans often rely on fortified soymilk as a source of calcium, vitamin B_{12}, and vitamin D, so check the label of the brand you prefer to make sure these important nutrients have been added.

Unflavored soymilk is mixed with a coagulant to make tofu in a process that is similar to making cheese. For best results, choose the right kind of tofu for the dish you'll be using it in. Silken tofu (often available in shelf-stable packaging) is best used for dishes where you want a creamy consistency—shakes, puddings, salad dressings, and pie fillings. Firm or extra firm tofu is a better choice for stir-fries and other dishes where you want the tofu to keep its shape. Once a package of refrigerated tofu is opened, any unused tofu should be refrigerated and covered with water. Shelf-stable tofu should be refrigerated after opening but does not need to be covered with water.

Tempeh, a popular addition to soups and casseroles, originated in Indonesia. Tempeh is made from whole soybeans that have been fermented, either alone or with a grain. Tempeh has a crumbly texture that some find reminds them of meat.

TVP is made from soy flour. It is often found in the bulk section of natural foods stores. TVP is sold in chunks and granules and may be flavored to taste like beef or chicken. TVP must be soaked in boiling water to rehydrate it. It can then be used in chili, sloppy joes, spaghetti sauce, and other recipes in place of ground beef.

Wheat Meat and Other Not Meats

If you've eaten in a vegetarian Chinese restaurant, you've probably eaten seitan. Seitan is made from gluten, the protein part of wheat. It has a chewy texture and can be baked, boiled, or stir-fried. Seitan is also called wheat meat and can be found in the refrigerated section of natural foods stores. You can also make your own seitan; a gluten flour mix makes it easy.

These days you can find a vegan version of almost any meat or seafood product. These "not meats" are often made from soy or seitan, although other beans and grains are sometimes used, especially in veggie burgers. Check labels—some have eggs, egg whites, or cheese added.

From Thanksgiving unturkey to Fourth of July veggie dogs, there are products for every occasion. These products are often high in protein and may be fortified with iron, zinc, or vitamin B_{12}. The downside is that they tend to be expensive.

Nut and Seed Butters

Nut and seed butters add protein, calories, and essential fats to vegan diets. Well-stocked stores feature almond butter, hazelnut butter, cashew butter, macadamia butter, and more. They can be used for sandwiches, to add richness to a smoothie, or to flavor soups, stews, and grain dishes. For those with nut allergies, try soy nut butter (made from roasted soybeans), sunflower seed butter, and tahini (sesame seed butter). See Chapter 22 for suggestions for making your own nut butter. Even if you still prefer peanut butter, check out some of the flavored peanut butters—from spicy to cinnamon-raisin.

Move Over Milk

Besides the previously mentioned soymilk, many other plant milks are available based on hemp seeds, almonds, oats, rice, and coconut. Which to choose is a personal preference, although if you are relying on plant milks as sources of key nutrients, be aware that not all are fortified and check the label to find one that meets your needs. Soymilk is highest in protein with 6–10 grams of protein in a cup. Oat milk and hemp milk have about half as much protein and rice, coconut, and almond milks only provide about 1 gram of protein per cup. Unflavored, original, or plain varieties of plant milks work best in savory dishes. Flavored milks (vanilla, chocolate, carob, and others) are sweeter and work in desserts and drinks.

Vegan cheese is typically made from rice, soy beans, peas, or nuts. It can be used in recipes that call for dairy cheese, but does not have the same nutritional profile. Some brands of vegan cheese do have calcium added. Most are quite low in protein. Grating or shredding vegan cheese helps it melt and combine with other ingredients.

Vegan yogurt can be found in the dairy case of supermarkets and natural food stores. Yogurt is commonly made from soymilk; coconut milk-based yogurt is a recent addition. Several brands of vegan yogurt are fortified with vitamins and minerals to resemble dairy yogurt.

ALERT

Packages of nondairy that say "lactose free" but do not say "vegan" or "casein-free" frequently contain casein, a protein that comes from cow's milk. Casein is what gives cheese its stretchy quality when melted. Cheese that contains casein is not vegan. Some brands of vegan cheese use other ingredients to mimic casein's stretchiness.

No Yolk (or White Either)

Commercial egg replacers containing various binding agents are often used to replace eggs in vegan baking. Ground flaxseeds can be blended with water and used as egg replacers. A tablespoon and a half of ground flaxseeds blended with ¼ cup of water can substitute for a large egg. You can purchase whole flaxseeds and grind them yourself or purchase them already ground (flaxseed meal). Opened packages of flaxseed should be stored in the freezer.

For Your Sweet Tooth

Vegans with a sweet tooth can find all sorts of vegan chocolates, baked goods, and frozen desserts at vegan bakeries or candy stores, natural food stores, and online. It's also easy to make your own desserts. See Chapter 22 for some ideas.

A Few Other Ingredients

Nutritional yeast is used in vegan recipes to add a cheese flavor. It can be sprinkled on popcorn or vegetables. This is not Brewer's yeast, which has a bitter flavor. You'll know it's nutritional yeast if you see pale yellow flakes or granules. One brand, Red Star's Vegetarian Support Formula nutritional yeast, is a reliable source of vitamin B_{12}. If you're buying nutritional yeast from the bulk food bin and relying on that to supply your vitamin B_{12}, check often to make sure the store is selling the vitamin B_{12}-rich form—you can definitely buy nutritional yeast that does not supply vitamin B_{12}.

If you have a favorite recipe that calls for honey or you like something sweet to add to herbal tea, you might try agave nectar. Agave nectar is a liquid sweetener produced from the juice of a succulent plant. Agave nectar mainly provides sugar and calories, so should be used in moderation.

Eating Organically Produced Foods

Many vegans choose to purchase at least some organically produced foods. If you're pregnant, you may be even more likely to seek out these foods, hoping to give your baby a healthy start. Just what is it that makes a food organic?

Organic foods are grown without using most conventional pesticides and fertilizers. A product that is identified as being organic is not produced by genetic engineering. Ionizing radiation and sewage sludge cannot be used in organic production or handling. Organic farming practices include soil and water conservation measures. Crop rotation, manure, and compost are used to improve the soil in place of using conventional fertilizers. Instead of using commercial insecticides or herbicides, organic farmers might use companion planting to discourage insects and mulch and hand weeding to control weeds.

Researchers continue to debate whether or not organically produced foods are more nutritious than conventionally grown products. Organic practices do benefit the environment as well as farm workers who are not exposed to potentially harmful pesticides and herbicides. Some people say that organic food tastes better.

The food label is where you can tell whether or not a product is organic. The USDA is responsible for the organic labeling program and allows one of three possible labels:

- Products labeled "100 percent organic" must contain only organically produced ingredients.
- Products labeled "organic" must have at least 95 percent of their ingredients organically produced.
- Products labeled "made with organic ingredients" must contain at least 70 percent organic ingredients.

Products that contain less than 70 percent organic ingredients can list individual ingredients as organic but cannot say that the product is organic.

Organic produce can be more costly than conventional produce. To reduce costs, buy locally and in season. If you can only afford to purchase some organic foods, focus on those where you don't remove the outer skin. Products where the thick peel or rind is removed before eating probably contain lower levels of pesticides than foods where the entire product, skin and all, is eaten. Think lemons versus apples, for example.

Eating Locally Grown Foods

Locally grown food has the advantage of being freshly picked. It has not been on a truck or in a warehouse for days before getting to the store. The farmer may only have to drive his beets five miles to the market rather than having them fly for thousands of miles from another country.

Another way to support your local farmer is to join a Community Supported Agriculture (CSA) farm. In the CSA model, a farmer sells shares in her farm. The shareholder receives a weekly supply of fruits and vegetables from the farm. You may go to a central location to pick up your share or it may be delivered to your house. Your CSA may include picking privileges—in season you can pick your own strawberries, green beans, cherry tomatoes, herbs, and more. Many CSAs feature organic produce. Although a CSA requires a considerable outlay ahead of the farming season, you then get many months of produce at no additional cost.

Once the baby comes, or if you have children already, trips to farms or farmers' markets are fun family outings that let your children see where their food comes from.

CHAPTER 10

Eating and Drinking Safely

You know what you need to eat, but did you know that there are some foods that should be avoided during pregnancy? Some of these foods (or beverages) contain substances that could be potentially harmful. Others have a higher likelihood of being contaminated with microorganisms that can cause foodborne illness. You may need to change some of your shopping habits and food prep techniques to reduce the risk of foodborne illness. Learning some of these safe food-handling habits now will help later when you're preparing baby or toddler meals.

Foodborne Illness

Every year, about one out of six Americans develops foodborne illness. Foodborne illness, also called food poisoning, is caused by eating food or drinking beverages that are contaminated with microorganisms—bacteria, viruses, or parasites. A foodborne illness can cause vomiting, diarrhea, and stomach cramps. Other symptoms are flu-like—fever, muscle aches, and headache.

Besides being an unpleasant experience, a foodborne illness is an especial concern in pregnancy. First of all, simply being pregnant increases your risk of developing a foodborne illness. Your immune system is not as active during pregnancy, so you're not as able to hold off bacteria and other contaminants. Your unborn baby's immune system is not mature enough to protect him from microorganisms.

FACT

Symptoms of foodborne illness can occur as soon as about twenty minutes after eating the contaminated food to as long as six weeks later. Most foodborne illnesses appear in one to three days, however, and last a few days. Some can leave you feeling ill for a longer time.

A second concern with a foodborne illness is that it can cause serious problems including miscarriage or premature delivery. Sometimes, even when your symptoms are mild, your baby can be negatively affected. Fortunately, there are some very specific steps you can take to reduce your risk of foodborne illness.

If, despite your best efforts, you think you have a foodborne illness, contact your health care provider immediately. Your blood may need to be tested to see what is causing your illness. You may need help staying hydrated if you have vomiting or diarrhea. Your doctor may prescribe an antibiotic that is safe to use in pregnancy. If you think your illness was from food you ate away from home, also contact the health department in your community. They can investigate the restaurant to reduce the risk of other people getting sick.

Foods to Avoid

Some foods should be completely off the menu in pregnancy because of their higher risk of contamination with microorganisms that could make you ill. Many of the foods on standard lists of foods to avoid are not vegan—raw eggs, undercooked meat, raw milk, soft cheeses, sushi, and some fish, for example. Vegans do have to be aware of some potential food-safety issues, however. Foods that should be avoided in pregnancy include raw sprouts of any kind and unpasteurized juice or cider. Raw sprouts are on the list of foods to avoid because potentially harmful bacteria can get into the sprout seeds before they are sprouted. Once bacteria are inside the seed's shell, it is very difficult to eliminate them. If you are eating out, ask that raw sprouts not be added to your sandwich or salad.

Fresh-squeezed juice, purchased in the supermarket or at a juice bar, may not be pasteurized. Pasteurization involves heating the juice to a temperature hot enough to reduce the number of microorganisms. Unpasteurized juices or cider should be avoided when you are pregnant.

The good news if you're vegan is that you don't have to worry about raw eggs in vegan cookie dough or raw fish in vegan sushi. Lunch meats often show up on the "to be avoided" lists, but vegan lunch meats are all right to eat.

If your kitchen is used to prepare meat, you'll need to take some precautions to make sure your food is not contaminated with microorganisms from the meat.

Kitchen Safety

Proper storage and handling of food, from the supermarket to your dinner table, is the best way to combat foodborne illness in your kitchen. On shopping day, make sure you check expiration labels before you buy. And because changes in storage temperature can breed bacteria in many foods, shop for refrigerated and frozen foods last and make sure they're the first items to be put away when you get home.

Safe Food Preparation

Your mom always told you to wash your hands before you started preparing foods and she was right. Hands need to be washed with soap and warm water before and after handling food, and after using the bathroom, changing a diaper, or handling a pet.

Food Safety if You Live with a Nonvegan

Even if you are a staunch vegan, you may be living with others who eat meat, fish, or poultry. Whether they prepare their own food or you make a meat meal for them and a vegan meal for yourself, it's important that everyone is clear on proper food handling.

ESSENTIAL

Interested in canning fruits and vegetables from your garden, CSA, or farmers' market? Make sure you preserve food safely. Visit the National Center for Home Food Preservation at *www.uga.edu/nchfp* for research-based information about methods of home food preservation. This website also offers USDA's *Complete Guide to Home Canning*, fact sheets, and consumer bulletins.

If you share a kitchen with someone who eats meat, be sure that all raw meat, poultry, and seafood are double-wrapped and stored in a separate area of the refrigerator to prevent any juices from contaminating other foods. These raw foods should also be isolated from other foods during meal preparation. Keep your refrigerator clean and wipe up spills immediately when they occur to discourage bacteria growth.

When someone in your household prepares raw meat, eggs, poultry, fish, or shellfish, all knives, dishes, cutting boards, food prep surfaces, and utensils that come in contact with the food need to be immediately and thoroughly cleaned. Try not to use the same cutting board for raw meat and fruits and vegetables. Hands should be washed with hot, soapy water. A clean set of utensils and serving dishes need to be used with the cooked food.

Fruit and Vegetable Safety

Fruits and veggies should also get a good cleaning. Thoroughly rinse everything you get from the produce stand and your own garden. Even veggies that are precut and packaged should be washed again before eating.

If you're doing your own vegetable or fruit gardening, do not use untreated manure, as it may harbor pathogens that could contaminate your fruits and vegetables.

Tofu Safety

Tofu is a perishable food, so make sure that the store where you purchase it keeps the tofu refrigerated and not tucked in with the vegetable display. Some markets or food co-ops may still sell bulk tofu in buckets of water—you select your tofu and place it in a container for purchase. There are many opportunities for this tofu to be contaminated, so avoid this kind of tofu when you are pregnant. Individually packaged tofu is a safer option, just be sure to use it before the expiration date. If you only use part of a package, place the remaining tofu in a clean container, cover with water, and refrigerate and use within a few days.

FACT

According to a scientific panel convened in 2006 by the National Institute of Environmental Health Sciences (NIEHS), the likelihood of use of soy products in pregnancy causing reproductive or developmental effects is of "negligible concern." Soy products, used in moderation, can make a significant nutrient contribution to a vegan diet.

Tofu that you plan to eat without cooking, for instance tofu used to make a smoothie or a sandwich spread, should be steamed 5–10 minutes before use. This extra step is usually not needed, but when you're pregnant, it's best to be safe.

Aseptically packaged tofu has been heat treated, so it does not need to be refrigerated before being opened. It also does not need to be steamed, even if you do plan to eat it without any additional cooking. Leftover aseptically packaged tofu should be refrigerated in a clean container and used within a few days.

Food Storage

When it's time to put away the leftovers, make sure you seal them up tightly and immediately refrigerate them. Leftovers should only be reheated once, to a temperature of 165°F (use a kitchen thermometer to check the temperature in the middle of the food).

Other Food Safety Issues

The bread that you bought a few days ago has blue fuzzy spots, the peaches you picked up for a pie are soft and have a white film, and the potatoes in the vegetable drawer have a greenish tinge. What's safe and what should be discarded?

Some molds can make you sick if you eat them. Some can cause breathing problems or allergic reactions. Not uncommonly, moldy food is also contaminated with bacteria.

Using foods shortly after purchase, checking for expiration dates, and keeping refrigerated foods covered are all ways to prevent mold growth. If you do discover moldy food, however, avoid smelling it to keep from inhaling the mold. Discard any food that is covered with mold and check any nearby items that the moldy food has touched. One moldy carrot can spread mold to other foods in the vegetable drawer.

Although it may seem simple to just cut out the moldy part of a food, this may not eliminate all parts of the mold. Molds send out "roots" that go below the food's surface. Getting rid of the mold can be difficult.

Small mold spots on firm fruits and vegetables with low moisture content (cabbage, broccoli stem, carrots) can be carefully cut off. Keep the knife out of the mold and cut off at least 1" around and below the mold spot. Soft fruits and vegetables with a high moisture content (peaches, tomatoes, cucumbers, strawberries) that are moldy should be discarded. Any other foods with mold including jelly, bread, leftovers, and veggie "meats" should be safely discarded.

Greenish potatoes can be contaminated with a toxic substance called solanine. Solanine can be fatal at high levels and can cause nausea, vomiting, and diarrhea. To be safe, discard potatoes with a greenish color or that taste bitter.

Dining Out

You can't ensure safe handling and preparation of your meals when you're not in control of the kitchen. But treating yourself to the occasional night out at a restaurant is perhaps even more important now that you're pregnant. When possible, go to restaurants you know and trust. When dining somewhere new, stick with safe menu choices that are less likely to harbor foodborne illness, such as pasta. Avoid anything sold off a cart or truck, and steer clear of eateries that look poorly kept and dirty (chances are the kitchen is, too).

When your meal is done, skip the doggie bag. Food should be refrigerated within two hours—counting from the moment the cook sticks it under the heat lamp. Allowing for a leisurely meal, a reasonably efficient wait staff, and travel time home from the restaurant, it's more than likely you won't make the cut off (unless you live above the restaurant or close to it)—giving your leftovers time to incubate bacteria.

Camping or Hiking

If you hike or camp, avoid drinking untreated water from streams or lakes or other bodies of water, no matter how clean the water looks. The parasite *Giardia duodenalis*, found in ponds and streams, is a common cause of waterborne illness. If you need to use water from a pond or stream, use purification techniques to kill *Giardia* and other parasites.

Boiling water is the surest way to purify it. If the water is muddy, let it stand to allow dirt to settle. Skim the clear water off the top, place it in a clean pot, bring it to a full boil, and continue to boil for 1 minute. At higher elevations, you will need to boil longer.

Water purification tablets, which usually contain iodine, halazone, or chlorine, are effective at killing most bacteria and viruses. They will not kill *Giardia*, however, so even if you use water purification tablets you will still need to filter the water through a 1-micron absolute or smaller filter. Bringing bottled beverages from home is another alternative.

Foods for hiking or camping should be nonperishable or kept chilled if they are perishable. Couscous, quick-cooking oatmeal, instant soup, powdered refried beans and hummus, nut butters, granola, and trail mix are all quickly prepared, nonperishable foods that are handy for outdoor trips. There's even a soy-based jerky that is shelf-stable.

Use the same safe food-handling techniques that you do at home. Be sure to wash hands well and to clean dishes using soap and hot water.

When the Power Goes Off

Whether it's an ice storm in January or a hurricane in August, there's a chance that you will lose electricity at some point in your pregnancy. It can be disconcerting to think of discarding everything in your refrigerator or freezer. That may or may not be necessary, depending on what the food is and how long the power is off.

As a rule of thumb, refrigerated food should be kept at a temperature of 40°F or colder and frozen food at or below 0°F. Keeping refrigerator and freezer doors closed as much as possible can help keep food at a safe temperature. An unopened refrigerator will keep food at a safe temperature for about four hours, according to the USDA. A full freezer will keep food at the recommended temperature for about forty-eight hours if the door remains closed; a half-full freezer will stay cold for about twenty-four hours.

Following a significant power loss, you will have to determine which foods are safe to keep. If power has been off for more than four hours, discard any perishable refrigerated food including tofu, soymilk or other milks, nondairy yogurts, mock meats, leftovers, and precut or prewashed packaged vegetables. Fresh, uncut fruits and vegetables can be kept. Never taste food to see if it is safe to eat—if in doubt, throw it out.

Frozen food that still contains ice crystals or is below 40°F is safe to refreeze, although there may be some loss of quality. If you share a refrigerator with a nonvegan and any food in the refrigerator or freezer has come in contact with raw meat juices, discard the food. For more information about disaster planning, see resources in Appendix A.

Alcohol

Drinking during pregnancy can cause problems. Whenever the mother has a drink, the alcohol goes into her bloodstream and passes through the placenta to her baby. The baby's liver is too immature to properly metabolize the alcohol, meaning it is more likely the alcohol will be harmful to the baby. In addition, drinking during pregnancy raises the risks for miscarriage or having a premature baby. See Chapter 2 for more information about the effects of alcohol during pregnancy.

In pregnancy, there is no known safe level of alcohol intake; all types of drinks present a risk. Complete avoidance of all alcohol—beer, wine, mixed drinks, liquor, and other alcoholic beverages—is safest for your baby. If, as you read this, you realize you have had alcohol since becoming pregnant, try not to obsess about it—resolve to avoid alcohol starting now. If you need help with an alcohol problem, talk honestly to your health care provider about treatment options. Local substance abuse programs are another source of help.

Caffeine and Artificial Sweeteners

Caffeine sources range from coffee and tea to cocoa, chocolate, some soft drinks, energy drinks, and some over-the-counter medicines. While moderate caffeine intake of about 200 milligrams a day (about 16 ounces of coffee) does not seem to increase the risk of miscarriage or premature birth, studies are conflicting and researchers cannot say with certainty what a safe level of caffeine in pregnancy is. Caffeine can also keep you from sleeping well, make nausea worse, and increase the number of trips you make to the bathroom.

You may be wondering about drinking diet sodas or using artificial sweeteners when you are pregnant. The FDA has determined that both aspartame (NutraSweet) and sucralose (Splenda) are safe for most people to use in moderation. The exceptions are anyone diagnosed with hyper phenylalanine (high levels of phenylalanine—a component of aspartame—in the bloodstream), with the genetic disease phenylketonuria (PKU), or with advanced liver disease.

Diet sodas can contain significant amounts of caffeine and can make you feel so full that you have little appetite for healthy foods. If you regularly drink diet sodas, consider cutting down or replacing them with water.

CHAPTER 11

Being Vegan in a Nonvegan World: Social Issues

You may have a large circle of like-minded vegan friends or you may not know any other vegans. Regardless, you're undoubtedly aware that it's not a vegan world. Social issues crop up—dinners with coworkers, holiday celebrations, visits to circuses and zoos. Being pregnant can complicate things. Will the baby be vegan? Can you be healthy and be vegan while you're pregnant? A few basic ideas will help you as you strive to be true to your vegan ideals.

Skeptical Friends

Your friends were used to your vegan diet when it was just you, but now you're going to be a mom. It seems like every time that you get together, your friends want to talk about your eating habits, and whether or not you're eating enough protein or whatever else your baby needs. Everyone seems to have a horror story about a friend of a friend who was vegan when she was pregnant and who ran into problems. How can you deal with all of this?

What's Really Going On?

Your friends care about you and want what's best for you. They need to know that you're thinking about good nutrition and getting what your baby requires. They want to be reassured that you have done your homework and that you know what you're doing. Your friends' eyes would probably start to glaze over if you walked them through every vitamin, mineral, and gram of protein you need and provided excruciating details about how you were going to do all of this. What's more important is that you calmly let them know that you're on top of things and that you're eating well, even if you are eating differently from them.

Options

If your friends are starting to get on your nerves with constant comments about your diet, you have several options. You may choose to use one or more of these possibilities, depending on the situation and how you otherwise feel about the friendship.

FACT

Although people may think that women are more often vegetarian, surveys such as those conducted by The Vegetarian Resource Group, typically find that about half of adult vegetarians are men. While vegetarians live everywhere, they're more likely to live in the western United States than in the Midwest.

Option One: Educate them. Remember, your friends are looking for reassurance that you're making good choices. Let them know that you've been reading about vegan pregnancy and that your health care provider is aware of your diet. You might mention positive things you're doing—taking a prenatal supplement, using fortified soymilk, cutting down on the junk food. Be ready to change the subject when necessary so that your eating habits do not become the sole topic of conversation.

Option Two: Agree to disagree. You've done your best to help your friend understand why you're eating the way you are and how you're making sure you're eating a healthy diet. In spite of everything, your friend continues to fret about your diet. A calm statement that lets your friend know that you appreciate her concern, you are convinced you're making good choices, and she's going to have to trust you on this one may be what's needed. Then change the subject.

Option Three: Let the friendship lapse. This may be the best choice if you find, despite your best efforts, that your eating habits are becoming the main focus of any encounter with a friend. Maybe this friendship will resume later, maybe it won't. In the meantime, be sure that you do have a support network of other friends.

Option Four: Seek out like-minded people. It may be time to look for some new friends. Maybe you'll find another vegan parent that you can commiserate with. Maybe you'll find a friend who's not vegan but has similar values to yours and who is comfortable with vegan diets.

Concerned Family Members

Just like your friends, your family may have gotten used to your vegan diet before you were pregnant. Now, however, they're expressing more concerns. They worry about protein and iron and whether you're eating enough. Actually, whether you're vegan or not, family members may seem to hover more when you're pregnant. If they weren't worrying about your diet, they might be worrying about how much work you're doing, or you continuing to exercise, or something else.

What's Really Going On?

Family members want what's best for you and for the baby. Just like friends, they want to know that you're making good choices. They may be concerned that you're not eating foods they think of as good foods for pregnancy—maybe foods that are traditional to their culture or that they ate when they were pregnant. They may worry that they won't be able to help you after the baby comes because they won't be able to make vegan food. They may be wondering if, a few years from now, they'll be able to make food for your children.

Making It Work

Option three for dealing with friends—letting the friendship lapse—is not really an option for family members. In order to figure out how to work with them, try to understand what they're really asking when they question your eating habits.

Some vegans have found that calmly providing supporting materials for their families to read is helpful. Perhaps you can photocopy a chapter or two from this book or show them a website from a reputable organization (see Appendix A). Find out what their concerns are and address them. Let them know that you've discussed your diet with your health care provider and with an RD, if you've done that.

Let your family know that you're not rejecting them, you just don't want to eat some of the foods that they eat. If they like to cook, this may be the time to share recipes with them or to invite them over so that you can show them how you make a simple dish or two. If your mom or mother-in-law collects cookbooks, give her a simple vegan cookbook—not because you expect her to become vegan but because you want her to be able to make vegan food if she wants to make food for you (and later for your child or children).

Nonvegan Partner

You're vegan; your partner isn't. Up until now, you've peacefully coexisted. Now, things are getting more confusing. How will the baby be raised? What will your child think if Mom eats one way and Dad another? There's no one-size-fits-all solution to these kinds of questions. As with other sensitive issues, your practices as a family will evolve and will be discussed over and over again.

More immediately, however, your partner may have the same concerns that friends and other family members have: is it safe for you to be vegan? Will the baby's nutritional needs be met? Similar strategies to those you're using for friends and family apply to your partner as well. You can provide factual information and reassurance. You can encourage your partner to discuss his concerns with your health care provider. Maybe you really haven't been eating that well and hearing your partner's concerns is the push you need to pay more attention. You can propose a consultation with an RD who can help you and your partner plan meals that will meet your needs.

What Would Emily Post Do? Vegan Etiquette

Whether it's the restaurant that thinks fish is a vegan option or the friends who tell you that the soup has "just a little chicken broth in it," vegans are faced with some challenging social situations. You're often walking the line between advocating for your needs and realizing that other people are clueless about what those needs are.

Dining Out

Here's the scenario: Your coworkers want to take you out to lunch to celebrate your pregnancy. They know you are vegan, but you really haven't told them about what that means. They are suggesting going to an Italian restaurant, thinking it will have food you can eat. When you check with the restaurant ahead of time, you learn that the pasta is made with eggs, all sauces have cheese in them, and that you can have steamed broccoli and a plain salad. What should you do? You know a good vegan restaurant, but you're afraid it may seem too strange to your very mainstream coworkers.

You have several options. You can go with your colleagues to the restaurant and smile while you eat a plate of lettuce. Your coworkers will probably feel badly and wonder why you're not eating something more. They may be concerned that they've offended you. It may be better to suggest another restaurant—either the vegan restaurant if your coworkers are adventurous types or a compromise place that has vegan options for you and familiar dishes for your officemates. A Chinese restaurant may be a good compromise if you feel confident it will have vegan foods. Let your colleagues know how much you appreciate the offer to go out to lunch, and that you don't expect them to know the ins and outs of your diet. Tell them that you checked with the restaurant they suggested and it has very little that you can eat, but you know another restaurant you think would work. Enjoy your lunch!

Family Events

Scenario: Your mom has been making your birthday cakes your whole life. You've recently become vegan and don't want to hurt her feelings, but you don't want her usual death-by-chocolate cake made with six eggs and two sticks of butter. What to do?

First of all, let your mom know how much you love her and how much you treasure the memories of all the cakes she's made for you. Talk to her well in advance of your birthday so she has time to work with you on possible ideas. Help her understand how important being vegan is to you and how that affects the kind of birthday cake you have.

ESSENTIAL

In place of cow's milk in vegan baking, you can use the same amount of plant-based milk. Milks can be soured to use in recipes calling for buttermilk by adding 1 tablespoon of lemon juice or vinegar to each cup of milk and letting it sit for a few minutes.

If your mom is open to it, suggest a good (and easy) vegan cake recipe that doesn't require a lot of exotic ingredients. See the dessert section of this book or vegan blogs or cookbooks for ideas. Don't be afraid to think outside the box. There's no rule that you have to celebrate a birthday with cake. If your mom is famous for another vegan dessert (maybe apple or peach pie), that might be a good choice for a birthday celebration. A store-bought cake is another idea. If you know a good vegan bakery, you could suggest that your family share a cake with you this year. This could be a good option if the idea of making a vegan cake is stressful for your mom.

Social Occasions

Here's the scenario: You've been invited to a baby shower for a friend. Your host has not mentioned any vegan food. In fact, you're not even sure the host knows you are vegan. Should you say something?

Put yourself in the host's position. Wouldn't you want to know if a guest had special needs? That's part of being a good host. As a good guest, you can make things easier for your host. Call ahead of time and explain your situation in very simple terms. Offer to bring a vegan dish to share. If the host tells you the menu, point out items that are vegan—maybe fruit salad or chips and salsa. If you're not sure there will be a lot of food you can eat and the host declines your offer to bring something, eat before you go and then fill a plate with food you can eat.

Holidays

Many family holidays revolve around food. And whether it's the Thanksgiving turkey, the Passover brisket, or the Fourth of July barbecue, the food is often not vegan.

QUESTION

Any ideas for a Thanksgiving entrée that everyone will like?
Thanksgiving is a harvest festival, so think of dishes that feature seasonal foods. Ideas include a winter squash stuffed with wild rice and vegetables; roasted vegetables; stuffed peppers; a vegan quiche; tamale pie; or curried chickpeas and potatoes. You could also go with a homemade or purchased vegan unturkey.

Your options include:

- Attend the family celebration and eat any vegan side dishes. Not a bad choice if you're comfortable with socializing with your family while they eat meat.
- Bring a vegan entrée to share. You'll still have to face the meat, but you'll have something more substantial to eat than side dishes. There's always the chance that other people will choose the vegan entrée over the meat entrée.
- Say you'll be able to come for dessert and bring a vegan dessert to share. You won't have to look at the meat, but you'll miss a part of your family gathering.
- Decide you'd prefer to have vegan holiday celebrations at your house and join your family for nonfood events or invite them to join you if they're okay with being vegan for the meal.

You have to decide which of these solutions, or others not listed, are most workable for your situation. Remember also that things change. Perhaps a relative's health issues will make your family more open to vegan celebrations in the future. Perhaps you'll feel less inclined to be at celebrations centered around meat when you have a young vegan. Do your best, and remember, it's not a vegan world.

Thinking Ahead

As you think ahead to having a child, you may be wondering how vegan families handle social events like birthday parties. Each family decides for itself how vegan their child or children will be. Some families send their child to parties with a vegan cupcake and a pint of vegan ice cream. Some families find that other parents are happy to make a vegan cake, especially if the circle of friends also includes children with dairy or egg allergies. Some families decide that it's all right for their child to eat vegetarian at birthday parties and stay vegan at home. What's right for your family may change over time, as your child becomes more aware of why he is vegan and is able to express his desires. There will be many situations where you'll have to make choices for your child.

Finding Other Vegans

You realize that you'd like to get to know other vegans. Maybe it's because socializing would be easier if you didn't have to bring a vegan entrée to make sure you have something to eat. Maybe you'd like to learn more about how other people do things or swap ideas for food or pregnancy or children. Maybe you'd just like to expand your circle of friends. Social networking sites can help, as can old-fashioned word of mouth.

Local Vegan Groups

Many communities have groups of vegans or vegetarians that meet regularly. Groups may have potluck dinners, host speakers, go out to a restaurant together, or plan for animal-related activities. To find a group in your area, look for calendar listings in the local newspaper. Check bulletin boards at natural food stores, vegetarian restaurants, and food co-ops. Contact area colleges or universities to see if there is a group on campus—they're often open to community members. National vegetarian organizations often have lists of local groups on their websites. You may see that a vegan cooking class is being offered at a store, restaurant, or school in your area. And, if there's not a local group, consider starting one.

National Vegan Groups

National vegan groups often hold conferences and exhibitions. If you live in or near a large city, you may be able to attend or volunteer at one of these events. Working on a committee makes it easy to meet other vegans. Some organizations sponsor weekend or week-long gatherings. For example, the North American Vegetarian Society (NAVS) holds Vegetarian SummerFest each year (see Appendix A for contact information).

Vegan Communities Online

From Facebook to vegan blogs, there are many opportunities to connect with other vegans online. Look for links on your favorite vegan websites or ask friends for suggestions. You can participate as much or as little as you choose.

Vegan Parent Groups

Some larger cities have vegan parent groups. Often these groups are a combination play group/support group. Ask around and check bulletin boards and newspaper calendar listings. The Vegetarian Resource Group (VRG) also has a parents' e-mail list for parents (including parents-to-be) who are raising a vegetarian or vegan child. To learn more, go to their website (*www.vrg.org*).

Will the Baby Be Raised Vegan?

Whether you and your partner are both vegans or you're the only vegan in the house, relatives and friends are likely to wonder how your child will be raised. Chances are if you and your partner are vegan, your baby will be raised as a vegan. Friends may challenge you for not giving your child a choice. Realistically, however, there are many decisions you make for your child—from what religion he practices to where he goes to preschool. When your child is old enough to accept responsibility for these types of decisions, they will be his to make. For now, it's up to you.

Nonvegan family members may be concerned that they won't be able to feed or care for a vegan child. Help them understand that you'll work with them to figure out solutions so they can pamper their vegan grandchild, niece, or nephew.

It gets tricky when one partner is vegan and one is not. You'll learn a lot about each other and about your relationship as you begin to discuss dietary choices for your child. Whether you choose to raise your child vegan, omnivore, vegan at home and nonvegan out of the home, or in some other fashion, the mutual love and respect that brought you together will help you as you assess each option and decide what will work for you.

Getting Help and Support

During or immediately after your pregnancy, you may need help from family or friends. You might be on bed rest or need meals after the baby is born. In an ideal world, you have dozens of vegan friends and family members who supply your every wish. More realistically, you'll need to work with nonvegans to help them help you.

As a first step, if someone offers to help, be clear about what you can't eat; don't expect people to know what vegan means. Provide recipe ideas and maybe even ingredients. Supplying a carton of soymilk, some vegan margarine, and your favorite brand of egg replacer can be a blessing to a nonvegan cook.

If your friends ask for menu suggestions, keep their food preparation skills in mind. Some people may be more comfortable with simple dishes like beans and rice, pasta salads, and lentil soup. Some friends may enjoy the challenge of using a vegan cookbook that you recommend. Some friends would be happy to pick up take-out, purchase prepared foods that meet your needs, or supply side dishes.

If you have time and energy, you can be proactive. Before the baby is born, make a double batch of some of your favorite recipes—one batch to eat right away and one to freeze for later. Doing this once or twice a week during the last trimester can give you several weeks' worth of vegan meals for when you and your partner want to focus on the baby and not on cooking.

CHAPTER 12

The First Trimester

During the first trimester, which lasts approximately fourteen weeks from the start of your last period, your baby's growth is amazing. By the end of your first month of pregnancy (four weeks since conception), your child's size will have increased 10,000-fold. In the second month, your baby will grow from about raisin size to almost the size of a grape. In the next month, baby will grow to over three inches long and weigh almost one ounce, about the size of a roll of Lifesavers.

Your Body This Trimester

From the first weeks where you may not notice much more than the absence of your monthly menstrual period to the end of the third month where you have a small pot belly, this first trimester is one of changes. By the end of this trimester, you will definitely feel pregnant. Your body is beginning to make the adjustments that are necessary to support your growing baby. From your tired and anxious mind to your busy bladder, all of your body's systems may seem to be in overdrive during the early days of pregnancy. Stay calm; all of these changes are normal and will become almost second nature as you progress through your pregnancy. It's an exciting time, too, especially at the end of this trimester, when you can hear your baby's heartbeat and perhaps even see him on ultrasound.

Your Body Changes

At the start of your pregnancy, you might not notice any immediate changes in your shape and size. The first thing you will notice is the absence of your monthly menstrual period—in many cases, this is what tipped you off to your pregnancy in the first place. Although you aren't menstruating, you feel slightly bloated, and your waistband may begin to feel a bit snug. On average, most women gain 1–4 pounds in the first trimester.

FACT

Some women experience minor vaginal blood flow or *spotting,* as the embryo implants itself into the uterine wall. Because of the timing—one week to ten days after ovulation—it's often mistaken for the beginning of the menstrual period. The spotting, which usually lasts only a day or two, is pink to brown and may be accompanied by minor cramps.

Your breasts may also start to increase in size, and the areolas around your nipples may enlarge and darken. No period? Bigger breasts? This baby is doing wonders for you already! Now for the cloud around that silver lining—fuller breasts are often more tender in pregnancy. A supportive sports bra can help.

You may also experience increased vaginal secretions similar to those you get premenstrually, another hormonal side effect. These typically last throughout pregnancy and may actually worsen in the third trimester, so stock up on panty liners now. Normal vaginal secretions in pregnancy are clear to white in color, mucus-like, and both odor and pain free. If you experience discharge that is thick, foul smelling, off-color, or accompanied by itching, blood, or pain, contact your health care provider immediately to rule out infection or other problems.

More Changes to Expect

Changes in skin and hair are common in pregnancy. Hair that was fine and thin may become thick and shiny during pregnancy, and that fabled pregnancy glow may actually be your flawless, blemish-free complexion. On the other end of the spectrum, acne problems and hair breakage and thinning may occur.

Chloasma (also known as melasma) may cause a mask-like darkening or lightening of your facial skin. Freckles and moles are prone to darkening, as are other pigmented areas of your skin. To minimize chloasma and other hyperpigmentation, use a good sunscreen (SPF 30 or higher) to cover exposed skin when you're out in the sun.

What You Feel Like

Building a baby is hard work, and even though it's early in the process, it isn't unusual to feel tired and rundown right now. If at all possible, try to grab a nap during the day. If that isn't feasible due to a full-time job or young children at home, make an early bedtime a priority. Although it may run contrary to your nature to be sleeping away the daylight hours, thinking of it as a naptime for baby might help. Once you start down the long road of sleepless nights that new motherhood brings, you'll be longing for the days of early bedtimes and frequent naps!

You may also find yourself spending more and more time in the bathroom. You are urinating more frequently due to high levels of progesterone, which relaxes your bladder muscles. Unfortunately, frequent urination is one symptom that will likely remain with you throughout pregnancy as your baby grows and the uterus exerts more and more pressure on your bladder.

Your cardiovascular system is undergoing big changes right now as it adjusts to meet baby's growing demand for the oxygen and nutrients your blood is carrying. Circulating pregnancy hormones dilate (or expand) your blood vessels to accommodate an eventual 50 percent increase in blood volume. Your cardiac output, a measure of how hard your heart is working to pump blood, increases 30–50 percent, whereas your blood pressure drops. This is why you may find yourself feeling faint. If you feel dizzy or lightheaded, sit or lie down on your side as soon as possible. Try not to lie flat on your back, particularly later in pregnancy, since the pressure your uterus places on two of the large blood vessels that help keep oxygen circulating to you and baby will actually make the dizziness worse.

ALERT

If episodes of fainting or dizziness persist or are accompanied by abdominal pain or bleeding, contact your health care provider immediately. They could be symptoms of ectopic (or tubal) pregnancy, a potentially fatal condition in which implantation occurs outside the endometrial lining of the uterus.

And then there's the most notorious of all pregnancy symptoms—morning sickness. Referred to by clinicians as nausea and vomiting of pregnancy (or NVP), up to 80 percent of women experience one or both of these symptoms at some point in their pregnancy. NVP can happen at any time and strikes with varying intensity. NVP and relief strategies are covered in depth later in this chapter.

Gas may become a source of discomfort and occasional embarrassment as well. Try to identify triggers and cut back on those foods. Beans, cabbage, broccoli, and carbonated drinks are common offenders. To keep problems at bay, try small, frequent snacks instead of large meals.

At the Doctor

Set up your first prenatal care visit as soon as you know you are pregnant. From now through the seventh month, you'll be seeing your provider on a monthly basis (if you are considered high risk, you may have more frequent appointments). If you're seeing a new doctor or midwife, expect your initial visit to be a bit longer than subsequent checkups since you'll be asked to fill out medical history forms and insurance paperwork. Some providers will send you these materials in advance so you can complete them at home. If you still haven't chosen a provider, now is the time to do so.

Your provider will ask questions about your health history and the pregnancy symptoms you have been experiencing. Make sure that you take advantage of this initial appointment to ask about issues that are on your mind as well. In addition to this interview time, you will undergo a thorough physical examination, give a urine sample (the first of many), and have blood drawn for routine lab work. If you haven't had a Pap smear within the last year, your provider may also perform this test. (For more on diagnostic and screening tests, see Chapter 13.)

ESSENTIAL

Remember, your partner is in this pregnancy, too. By all means, bring him to the doctor with you. In addition to providing moral support, he probably has just as many questions about the baby as you do. He can also help you remember the things your provider tells you that seem to promptly exit your brain as you leave the examining room.

Your provider will probably supply you with educational brochures and pamphlets on prenatal care, nutrition, office policies, and other important issues. There will be a lot of new information to absorb, so don't feel as though you have to study everything on the spot. However, do take everything home so you can read and refer to it later. Start a folder or notebook for keeping pregnancy information together. Add a pad of paper so you can jot down any questions for your provider.

When to Call the Doctor, Day or Night

At your first appointment, your provider may discuss how patient phone calls are handled both during the day and after hours. Frequently, obstetrical practices use a triage system where the receptionist or intake coordinator answers and prioritizes calls and has a nurse, midwife, or physician return them in order of urgency. If your doctor is in the office and you feel more comfortable speaking with her directly, be sure to make your preference known when you call.

Usually an answering service will pick up after-hours calls and will page the doctor or midwife on duty, who will then return your call. In most group practices, providers usually take turns covering nights and weekends, so you will get a call back from the on-call practitioner. If you aren't given any guidelines for reaching staff after hours, make sure you ask. Call your doctor immediately if you experience any of the following symptoms:

❑ Abdominal pain and/or cramping

❑ Fluid or blood leaking from the vagina

❑ Abnormal vaginal discharge (foul smelling, green, or yellow)

❑ Painful urination

❑ Severe headache

❑ Impaired vision (spots, blurring)

❑ Fever over 101°F

❑ Chills

❑ Excessive swelling of face and/or body

❑ Severe and unrelenting vomiting and/or diarrhea

Some women hesitate to pick up the phone for fear they're being oversensitive or a hypochondriac. While a good dose of common sense should be used in contacting your doctor after hours, in most cases better safe than sorry applies. Learn to trust your instincts; if something just doesn't feel right to you, make the call.

Get the Most Out of Monthly Checkups

Bring along that list of questions that have come to you and your partner since your last visit. Make sure your questions are answered before you leave; although it's nice to be asked if you have any concerns, in the busy atmosphere of an obstetrical practice your provider may occasionally forget.

Never feel like you're being pushy or overbearing (remember, you're leading this team). In most cases, he will do what he can to educate you and reduce any anxieties. If he doesn't, it's never too late to find someone who will.

Baby's Heartbeat

Hearing the steady woosh-woosh of your baby's heart for the first time is one of the most thrilling and emotional moments of pregnancy. Your chance at first contact happens the third month, as your provider checks for the fetal heartbeat using a small ultrasound device called a *Doppler* or *Doptone*. Make sure your husband or partner makes this month's prenatal appointment. You're both in for a treat as you begin to experience the sights and sounds of your growing child.

On Your Mind

Pregnancy, particularly a first pregnancy, is a time of great anticipation as you head into uncharted waters. Pregnancy is also a precursor to one of the biggest life-changing events there is—the arrival of a baby—and that alone is enough to stir up new and unexpected feelings.

Now that you've officially started this journey, you may be surprised to find yourself filled with conflicting emotions.

Elation, Excitement, and Anxiety

You may be thrilled beyond belief. You are creating a new and unique life of boundless potential. As a family, you will share your hopes, dreams, knowledge, and love. This is one of the most important tasks—and special experiences—of your life. So excitement is the order of the day.

Coupled with the excitement are concerns. Worries about the baby's health and the possibility of miscarriage are common fears early in pregnancy. If you've had a previous miscarriage, you may be walking on eggshells trying to second-guess every move you make. The good news is that knowing your history of miscarriage, your provider is following your progress closely.

Although easier said than done, letting go of your anxieties is the best thing for you and your baby right now. Try designating a certain area of your home, like your bedroom, a worry-free zone, and then stick to a vow to let your anxieties go when you are in that space. Use sounds, sights, and smells to make it as comfortable and relaxing as possible. An aromatherapy candle you like, soft music or nature sounds, and some soothing scenery in the form of photographs and posters can do wonders for your state of mind.

You might also be concerned about your ability to provide for and care for your child. It's important to remember that good parents learn with experience and by the experiences of others. The very fact that you're reading this book and getting regular prenatal care shows that you want the best for your baby. By the time your baby arrives, you'll be surprised at how much you will have learned in the relatively short period of nine months.

Emotional Health

The hormonal changes that occur in pregnancy can have you feeling weepy one minute, irritable the next, and elated the next. If you're normally the even-keeled type, these emotional flip-flops can be downright alarming. You aren't losing control or losing your mind, you're just experiencing the normal mood swings of pregnancy. Although this emotional lability may continue throughout pregnancy, it is typically strongest in the first trimester as you adjust to hormonal and other changes.

Stress and Stress Management

It's easy to get stressed out over what may seem like an overwhelming amount of preparation for your new family member. Your body is already working overtime on the development of your child; try to keep your commitments and activities at a reasonable level to prevent mental and physical overload.

Controlling outer stress is especially important when your pregnant body is under the physical stress of providing for a growing baby. And added psychological stress can make the discomforts of pregnancy last longer and feel more severe.

Effective stress management involves finding the right technique for you. Relaxation and meditation techniques (for example, progressive muscle relaxation, yoga), adjustments to your work or social schedule, or carving out an hour of me time each evening to decompress are all ways you can lighten your load. Exercise is also a great stress-control method, but be sure to get your doctor's approval regarding the level of exercise appropriate for you.

Forgetfulness

Have you walked around looking for your sunglasses for twenty minutes before finding them on your head? Like any mom-to-be, you've got a lot on your mind. That alone may have you forgetting details that used to be second nature and misplacing items. Although researchers have looked at the problem of memory impairment in pregnancy, there hasn't been a clear consensus on the definitive cause. Pregnancy hormones, sleep deprivation, and stress have all been suggested as possible culprits. Think about carrying a small notebook with you as a memory crutch. This can keep you from losing your mind—and your car.

Morning Sickness

Your stomach flutters, then lurches. Then you run for the bathroom for the fifth time today. Sound familiar? NVP is arguably the most debilitating and prevalent of pregnancy symptoms. While most women find that NVP symptoms subside or stop as the first trimester ends, for some they continue into the second and even third trimester. If you're having twins or more, your NVP may also be longer and more intense.

The exact cause of NVP has not been pinpointed, but theories abound. Some possible culprits: the human chorionic gonadotropin (hCG) hormone that surges through your system and peaks in early pregnancy; a deficiency of vitamin B_6; hormonal changes that relax your gastrointestinal tract and slow digestion; and immune-system changes. Another hypothesis is that morning sickness is actually a defense mechanism that protects both mother and child from toxins and potentially harmful microorganisms in food. No matter what the trigger, it's a miserable time for all.

Remedies and Safety

The following treatments have met with some success in lessening symptoms of NVP in clinical trials. Speak with your health care provider before adding any new supplements to your diet.

- **Ginger.** Ginger snaps and other foods and teas that contain ginger may be helpful in settling your stomach.

- **Acupressure wristbands (Sea-Bands).** Sometimes used to ward off motion and seasickness, these wristbands place pressure on what is called the P6 or Nei-Kuan acupressure point. Available at most drugstores, they are an inexpensive and noninvasive way to treat NVP.
- **Vitamin B$_6$.** This supplement has reduced NVP symptoms in several clinical trials. It has been suggested that NVP is a sign of B$_6$ vitamin deficiency.

ALERT

Kava-Kava, licorice root, rue, Chinese cinnamon, and safflower are just a few of the many botanical remedies known to be dangerous in pregnancy. Don't pick up that supplement or cup of herbal tea without asking your health care provider first.

Other coping methods that women report as helpful include:

- **Eating smaller, more frequent meals.** An empty stomach produces acid that can make you feel worse. Low blood sugar causes nausea as well.
- **Choosing proteins and complex carbohydrates.** Protein-rich foods (tofu, beans) and complex carbs (baked potato, whole-grain breads) are good for the two of you and may calm your stomach.
- **Eating what you like.** Most pregnant women have at least one food aversion. If broccoli turns your stomach, don't force it. The better foods look and taste, the more likely they are to stay down.
- **Sticking to bland foods if you find fatty or spicy foods distasteful.** Traditional comfort foods nourish many women suffering through morning sickness; staples like noodle soup, plain rice and pasta, and baked or mashed potatoes can be a filling way to get needed calories.
- **Drinking plenty of fluids.** Don't get dehydrated. If you're vomiting, you need to replace those lost fluids. Some women report better tolerance of beverages if they are taken between meals rather than with them. Turned off by water and juice right now? Try juicy fruits

like watermelon and grapes instead or make your own juice bars by freezing fruit juice in a mold.

- **Brushing regularly.** Keeping your mouth fresh can cut down on the excess saliva that plagues some pregnant women. Breath mints may be helpful, too.

- **Asking for help.** Preparing meals when you're not feeling well can be even more challenging than eating them, so try to get help in the kitchen from your spouse or significant other, if possible. If not, stock up on foods that require minimal prep work, such as frozen entrées and canned soups, so you can eat with little effort.

- **Talking to your provider about switching prenatal vitamins.** If it makes you sick just to look at your vitamin, perhaps a chewable or other formulation will help. Iron is notoriously tough on the stomach, so your provider might also recommend a supplement with a lower or extended release amount. And if you can't keep your vitamin down no matter what you try, your doctor may suggest foregoing it for now until your NVP has passed.

When It May Be More than Morning Sickness

When your body can't get what it needs from food to keep things running, it will start to metabolize stored fat for energy. This condition, called *ketosis*, generates a substance called *ketones* that circulate in your bloodstream and can be harmful to your fetus. Your provider may test your urine for ketones if you're having severe and persistent nausea and vomiting.

ESSENTIAL

Put together a morning sickness survival kit for the car. Items to include: wet wipes, tissues, small bottle of water, travel-sized toothbrush and toothpaste, breath mints, graham or soda crackers, and a bundle of large freezer-grade zipper-lock baggies. For longer trips, a cell phone and a *just-in-case* change of clothes are a necessity.

A small percentage of pregnant women (0.3–3 percent) experience a severe form of morning sickness called *hyperemesis gravidarum*. If you can't keep any food or fluids down, are losing weight, and are finding it impossible to function normally, you may be in this category.

Even though hospitalization is sometimes required for hyperemesis gravidarum, the good news is that the treatment—intravenous fluids to restore fluid and electrolyte balance and, in some cases, antiemetics (drugs to stop vomiting)—is relatively simple. If you are prescribed antiemetics, talk with your doctor about the safety data on the drug you are prescribed and any potential effects on the fetus.

If you're dealing with morning sickness, eating healthfully (and keeping it down) is a particular challenge. Your stomach will have definite opinions on what it will and will not tolerate; when you're feeling nauseous, let it guide you. Stick to what works—even if it's the same thing three times daily. Morning sickness won't last forever, and prenatal vitamins will help even out your nutrient intake while you get through this difficult period. Don't worry if you don't gain weight in the first trimester due to morning sickness; it's more important to have weight gain in the following trimesters.

CHAPTER 13

The Second Trimester

Welcome to the second trimester, what many women consider "the fun part." Your energy is up and your meals are staying down. You're looking pregnant, so take advantage of designated close-in pregnancy parking spaces without feeling guilty. You and your baby are in the midst of a period of rapid growth now, so it's not surprising that you're feeling tired—pregnancy is hard work! Treat yourself to naps and sleeping in on the weekend. Remember, at the end of this trimester, you'll be more than halfway there!

Your Body This Trimester

At the beginning of this trimester, you'll probably actually sense your child inside of you—a humbling and life-affirming experience. By the end of the trimester, you may be seeing fetal movement across your abdomen as baby gets comfortable in her shrinking living space. As your uterus expands, your center of gravity shifts, so be careful if you're walking in slippery or icy conditions.

Your appetite is likely to pick up early in the second trimester. That's fortunate, because you'll gain about 60 percent of your total pregnancy weight (11–15 pounds) in this trimester.

Movement!

Think that ultrasound was exciting? Just wait until you feel your little gymnast stretch and push inside of you for the first time. By week 19, most women have felt that distinctive first flutter, often described in terms of butterfly wings or bubbles.

ALERT

> Once baby starts moving regularly, on average, you should feel five or more movements each hour. Three or fewer movements or a sudden decrease in fetal activity could be a sign of fetal distress, so if you notice either, call your provider to follow up as soon as possible.

You'll quickly discover that your baby is already establishing behavioral patterns. When you're up and about, she can be rocked to sleep by your movements. Then when you lie down and try to take a rest, she wants to get up and groove. Is your partner having trouble getting a hand on your stomach in time to feel the fetal kung fu? Have him stand by during a lying-down time and see whether he catches a kick or two.

Stretch Marks

The skin of your belly is stretching, tightening, and most likely itching like crazy. A good moisturizing cream (look for one that does not contain animal products and that was not tested on animals) can relieve the itching and keep your skin hydrated, although it won't prevent or eliminate stretch marks. Whether or not you develop stretch marks is largely a matter of genetics, although factors such as excessive weight gain and multiples' gestations increase your odds of having them.

QUESTION

I think I'm getting varicose veins! What can I do to stop the discomfort?
Increased blood volume in pregnancy can damage the valves that regulate blood flow up through the blood vessels of the legs. The result is pooled blood in the vein and that telltale squiggly red or blue line. Supportive stockings and resting on your left side can relieve any leg soreness.

The red, purple, or whitish striae are created by the excess collagen your body produces in response to rapid stretching of the skin. They may appear on your abdomen, breasts, or on any other blossoming body part right now. Don't be too alarmed, since striae typically fade to virtually invisible silver lines after pregnancy.

Aches and Pains

You may start to feel occasional discomfort in your lower abdomen, inner thighs, hips, and lower back. A combination of the increasing work muscles in these areas are doing and hormonal effects lead to these aches. Pelvic tilt exercises are useful for relieving aches.

The pelvic tilt can be performed while standing against a wall, although it might be more comfortable done on hands and knees. Keep your head aligned with your spine, pull in your abdomen, tighten your buttocks, and tilt your pelvis forward. Your back will naturally arch up. Hold the position for three seconds, and then relax. Remember to keep your back straight in this neutral position. Repeat the tilt three to five times, eventually working up to ten repetitions.

To help with lower back pain, practice good posture when sitting or standing. Avoid sudden twists and turns and put the high heels away for now. Some women find that using a low stool to rest their feet when sitting helps. If you must stand for long periods, alternate resting each foot on a step. Some stretching and flexibility exercises may be in order. Check with your health care provider for approval and recommendations; if the pain is troublesome enough or if you have a history of back problems, he may suggest a physical therapist to work with.

ALERT

If your abdominal and/or back pains are severe or accompanied by fever, vomiting, vaginal bleeding, or leg numbness, call your health care provider immediately. Most minor back pain in pregnancy is completely normal, but in severe cases it can also be a sign of preterm labor, kidney infection, or other medical problems.

You may also notice leg cramps. Stretching out your calf muscles can often quash a cramp. A number of studies have found that magnesium supplements can reduce the incidence of cramps in some women. Check with your health care provider to see what she suggests. Dietary sources of magnesium include whole grains, dried beans, soy products, nuts, and leafy greens.

If your leg pain is accompanied by swelling, redness, and skin that is warm to the touch, call your health care provider to report your symptoms. You could be experiencing deep vein thrombosis (DVT), a blood clot in your leg that impedes circulation and has the potential to embolize or break off and block a major blood vessel. Pregnant women are more likely to develop DVT; however, DVT itself is relatively rare, occurring in less than one of every 1,000 pregnancies.

At the Doctor

Beyond the usual weight and measure routine, your doctor may administer a glucose challenge test (GCT) between weeks 24 and 28. Women who have chosen to take an alpha-fetoprotein (AFP)/triple/quad test will have their blood drawn sometime between week 15 and 18. You can read more about these tests later in this chapter.

Premature Labor

Delivery of your baby after week 20 and before week 37 of pregnancy is considered preterm or premature. In cases of very early preterm labor where fetal lung maturity hasn't been established, your provider will probably try to delay the delivery for as long as possible. Preemies can suffer from a wide range of physical, neurological, and developmental difficulties, so any extra time spent in the womb is beneficial.

If you experience any of the following warning signs of preterm labor, call your health care provider immediately. If you are out of town or unable to get in touch with her for any reason, go directly to the nearest hospital emergency room. With prompt action, it may be possible to delay your labor until your unborn child has adequate time to develop.

Symptoms include:

- Painful contractions at regular intervals
- Abdominal cramps
- Lower backache
- Bloody vaginal discharge
- Stomach pain
- Any type of fluid leak from the vagina, large or small

Preterm labor may be halted by bed rest, drugs that stop contractions, and intravenous hydration. Depending on your medical history and the stage of your pregnancy, you may be hospitalized. Home bed rest may also be prescribed, and you might be required to hook up to a fetal monitor on a regular basis. If preterm labor occurs between 24 and 34 weeks, corticosteroids may be administered to hasten fetal lung development, as well.

On Your Mind

It may seem as if you're on an emotional roller coaster. One day you're ready to conquer the world and the next you feel irritable and overwhelmed. Your emotions are very close to the surface. Try to defuse difficult situations by having an action plan for coping. And don't hesitate to accept small favors such as a closer parking space or a cushy chair in the conference room.

Irritability

Because of all the added demands on your body, mind, and emotional equilibrium, you could be finding yourself short on patience these days. Pregnancy is the perfect excuse for steering clear of people who—let's face it—are just plain annoying. Avoidance isn't the ultimate answer, of course, but during this crucial time in which your emotional and physical balance are so important, it's a good solution for taking care of the little things and keeping your sanity intact.

QUESTION

Can the seat belt in my car hurt the baby?
Definitely continue to buckle up for safety throughout your pregnancy. The lap belt should fit snugly under your belly bulge, and the shoulder belt should be positioned between your breasts. Don't worry about the belt hurting the baby; the uterus and fluid-filled amniotic sac are excellent shock absorbers.

If family and friends are getting your ire up as well, it might be a sign that you are feeling overwhelmed and undersupported. Take a look at what's really getting to you. Remember that you aren't in this alone. If you're single, enlist family or close friends to help out. And if you are married but still aren't getting the help and support you need from your husband, ask for it. Although it's nice when others anticipate your needs and pitch in voluntarily, they may be wrapped up in their own preparations and anxieties about the new family addition. Don't feel guilty about reminding them that their help is needed.

Getting Enough Sleep

Perhaps it's nature's way of preparing you for the sleepless nights to come, but your growing belly and the pushes and prods of your little one are making it increasingly difficult to get the requisite eight or more hours of peaceful slumber. Sleep is essential to your mental and physical fitness right now, not to mention that of your unborn child. Make your best effort to rest often and rest well.

- Make a regular bedtime and stick to it.
- If your schedule permits, try to make up your sleep deficit with a daytime nap.
- Experiment with a foam egg-crate cushion on your mattress or a body pillow for extra padding.
- Make the bathroom the last stop before bed.
- Stay away from caffeine (it isn't the best thing for you right now, anyway).
- Don't exercise for up to three hours before bedtime.

Exercise

Don't avoid the gym, pool, or other favorite places to exercise just because you're pregnant. Exercise will not only make you feel better, it can tone muscles that will be getting a workout in labor and delivery.

ALERT

Certain activities are definitely off limits during pregnancy. These include scuba diving, water skiing, downhill snow skiing, and contact sports. Gymnastics and horseback riding should be avoided because of the increased risk of falling. In addition, proceed with caution when participating in potentially high-impact activities like tennis, volleyball, and aerobics.

Exercise guidelines issued by ACOG recommend thirty minutes of moderate exercise activity daily for women who are pregnant (excluding high-risk pregnancies). Swimming and walking are recommended forms of exercise. More strenuous exercise (like jogging, biking, and some sports) may be fine during pregnancy if you are physically fit and exercised before you were pregnant. All pregnant women, especially those in high-risk pregnancies and those who were inactive prior to pregnancy, should speak with their physician about exercise options.

Exercise doesn't have to be complicated, expensive, or technically difficult. It can be as simple as tossing a ball with the kids in the backyard, taking the dog on a brisk walk each evening, or swimming or even walking laps in the local pool. Thirty minutes of regular, heart-pumping activity started and capped off by a good stretching routine is all it takes to benefit you and baby. Above all, make sure it's an activity you enjoy or do in good company, so you will look forward to it.

If you thrive on routine and feel more likely to get moving if you have a set schedule, check out your local YMCA, hospital, or community center for a prenatal exercise class. Water exercise programs are also a good low-impact way to get fit. Even if your class is tailored toward moms-to-be, check with your doctor first.

Precautions

While exercise can be a boon to your body and baby, there are basic steps you should take to stay safe. First and foremost, run your routine by your provider to get a medical stamp of approval. If you're new to working out, start slowly. Be attuned to your body's signals and stop immediately if you experience warning signs such as abdominal or chest pain, vaginal bleeding, dizziness, blurred vision, severe headache, or excessive shortness of breath.

Dress in supportive, comfortable clothing that breathes well and braces your belly and other parts of your expanding anatomy. If your feet have swollen past the comfort level of your old gym shoes, invest in a bigger pair. Drink plenty of caffeine-free fluids before, during, and after your workout to remain well hydrated, and try to work out in a climate-controlled environment to avoid a sharp rise in core body temperature, since overheating can be hazardous to a developing fetus.

Kegels are one exercise every pregnant woman should know and practice. They strengthen the pelvic muscles for delivery and can improve the urinary incontinence (or dribbling) that some women experience in pregnancy. What's a Kegel? Tighten the muscles you use to shut off your urine flow, hold for four seconds, and relax. You've just done your first Kegel. Try to work up to ten minutes of Kegels daily.

Screening and Diagnostic Tests

You'll be poked, prodded, swabbed, scraped, and scanned throughout your pregnancy. All these tests have a purpose, of course—a healthy mom and baby. Prenatal tests elicit the full spectrum of maternal emotions, from calm reassurance to amusement to anxiety and fear of the unknown. Knowing what to expect can make these exams more comfortable.

Urine Tests

You'll be giving a urine sample at each prenatal visit for urinalysis. Your provider's office or lab will test your urine for ketones, protein, and glucose, and may also check for the presence of any bacteria. These tests are simple; a strip of chemically treated paper is dipped in your urine sample. Your urine is tested for ketones as indicators of either insufficient nourishment due to severe nausea and vomiting or poorly controlled gestational diabetes. The test for protein in your urine is a check for preeclampsia, urinary tract infection (UTI), and renal (kidney) impairment. Glucose (or sugar) in the urine (called glycosuria) can be a sign of GDM. It's normal to spill a small amount of sugar into the urine in pregnancy, but consistently high levels along with other risk factors raise a red flag that GDM may be present. Positive results on any of these tests usually call for additional testing.

Blood Work

Early in pregnancy, and possibly in the second and third trimesters, your blood hemoglobin level will be measured to check for iron-deficiency anemia. Blood tests can also screen for inherited anemia in at-risk populations. For example, couples of African, Caribbean, Eastern Mediterranean, Middle Eastern, and Asian descent are at risk for sickle cell anemia. Families of Greek, Italian, Turkish, African, West Indian, Arab, or Asian descent may be screened for the thalassemia trait.

Your blood type and Rhesus (or Rh) factor will be determined at your first prenatal visit. An Rh factor is either positive or negative. If your Rh is positive, no treatment is necessary. If you are Rh negative and your partner is Rh positive, you are at risk for Rh incompatibility with the blood type of your baby. Rh incompatibility can occur when your unborn baby is Rh positive. If some of the baby's blood enters your bloodstream, your body may produce antibodies against the baby's blood, causing her to have severe anemia. When this happens, your immune system may try to fight off the baby as an intruder, causing serious complications. If caught early on, however, the disorder can be treated effectively later in pregnancy

QUESTION

I'm forty. What are my chances of an uncomplicated pregnancy?
Women over age thirty-five have a higher risk for developing diabetes, high blood pressure, and placental problems in pregnancy. There is also an increased risk of having a baby with a chromosomal disorder. The good news is that proper prenatal care can greatly reduce your risk of these complications.

Blood tests also determine whether or not you are immune to German measles (rubella), a disease that can cause birth defects, especially if you contract it during the first trimester. An HIV, hepatitis B, and syphilis test may also be done on your blood.

Typically between weeks 24 and 28 of pregnancy, you will be given a glucose challenge test as a screening tool for GDM. The test requires you to drink 50 grams of a glucose solution, a sugary flavored drink usually called glucola. One hour later, blood will be drawn and your blood glucose levels will be measured. If your results exceed the guidelines your doctor has established, further testing will be necessary.

Swabs and Smears

Unless you've had one in the twelve months leading up to conception, your provider will give you a Pap smear at your initial prenatal visit. Swabs of both the rectum and the vagina will be done at weeks 35–37 of gestation to check for Group B streptococcus (GBS). If a pregnant woman tests positive for this bacterium that can cause serious infections in a newborn, she is usually prescribed intravenous antibiotics during labor and delivery. Depending on your medical history and perceived risk factors, your provider may also test for chlamydia, gonorrhea, or bacterial vaginosis by means of a vaginal swab sample.

Ultrasounds

The eagerly awaited ultrasound gives you your first glimpse at your little one and lets your practitioner assess the baby's growth and development. It may also be used to diagnose placental abnormalities, an ectopic pregnancy, certain birth defects, or other suspected problems. There are two types of ultrasound scans: the transabdominal, which scans through your abdomen, and the transvaginal, which scans directly into your vagina. In very early pregnancy, the technician may opt for the vaginal approach, which means that the transducer (or handheld wand) will be inserted into your vagina. However, abdominal ultrasounds are the most common since most ultrasounds take place in the second or third trimesters.

ESSENTIAL

If your fetus isn't feeling coy on ultrasound day, a sonogram taken after sixteen weeks may reveal its sex. A sighting of a little girl's labia (visible as three parallel lines) or a boy's penis can provide a fairly positive ID, but keep in mind that ultrasound is not foolproof and parents have been surprised in the delivery room.

An ultrasound typically takes no longer than a half hour to perform. If you are in the first half of your pregnancy, you will probably be instructed to drink plenty of water prior to the exam and refrain from emptying your bladder. This is probably the most difficult part of the test. The extra fluids help the technician visualize your baby.

Many obstetricians order ultrasounds as a matter of routine. Some do one at the first visit to check for correct dates and viability, with the rationale that it may save them from questioning gestational dates later on (since dating is more accurate when done in the first trimester). Others will recommend a sonogram at around week 20 to examine the fetal anatomy and ensure the pregnancy is progressing normally.

AFP/Triple or Quad Screen Test

The maternal serum AFP test, usually administered between weeks 15 and 18, is a blood test used to screen for chromosomal irregularities such as trisomy 18 and trisomy 21 (Down syndrome), and also for neural tube defects. It can also indicate the presence of twins, triplets, or more. A more precise version of the AFP called the triple-screen test (or AFP-3) measures levels of hCG and estriol, a type of estrogen, as well as AFP. The quad-test, an even more sensitive marker of chromosomal problems, assesses all three of these substances plus inhibin A.

Amniocentesis

An amniocentesis involves two critical undertakings: a needle being inserted through the abdomen and breeching your baby's watery environment. It does carry some risk of complications, including a slight chance of miscarriage. However, the amnio is one of the best tools available for diagnosing genetic disorders and chromosomal abnormalities. An amniocentesis is typically performed in the second trimester sometime between weeks 15 and 20 of pregnancy, although a later amnio may be done depending on the indication.

FACT

The CDC estimates the chance of miscarriage following an amnio at somewhere between 1 in 400 and 1 in 200, and the risk of uterine infection at less than 1 in 1,000. There is also a slight risk of trauma to the unborn baby from a misplaced needle or inadvertent rupture of the sac.

Your provider may suggest you meet with a genetic counselor prior to having an amniocentesis performed to weigh the risks versus the benefits of the procedure, given your specific medical background and family history.

After the amnio procedure, the baby will be monitored by ultrasound and will have his heart rate checked for a few minutes to ensure that everything is okay. Minimal cramping may follow the procedure. You will be advised to restrict strenuous exercise for a day (no step aerobics and no sex), although other normal activity should be fine. If in the days following amnio you experience fluid or blood discharge from the vagina, let your provider know as soon as possible.

Chorionic Villus Sampling (CVS)

CVS is performed in the first trimester (usually between weeks 10 and 12) to assess chromosomal abnormalities and hereditary conditions in the unborn baby. Your provider will use ultrasound guidance to insert a catheter into the placenta, either through the cervix or through a needle injected into the abdomen. The catheter is used to extract a biopsy (or sample) of the tiny chorionic villi, the fingers of tissue surrounding the embryo that are the beginnings of the placenta. The villi are a genetic match for the baby's own tissue.

Slight cramping and spotting is normal after the procedure, and you will probably be advised to indulge in some rest and relaxation for the remainder of the day. If bleeding continues, is excessive, or is accompanied by pain or fever, call your practitioner immediately.

ESSENTIAL

Some studies suggest that the experience and associated skill level of the physician performing a CVS or amniocentesis can make a big difference in the risk of complications. Many physicians will refer you to a specialist for just this reason. If your provider is performing the procedure, ask for an estimate of how many amnios or CVS procedures he has performed.

CVS has several benefits over amnio. It can be performed earlier (first trimester as opposed to second) and the results are available much faster (five to seven days for preliminary CVS results versus ten to fourteen days for amnio). However, the risk of miscarriage is higher with CVS—between 1 in 200 and 1 in 100 will experience miscarriage after the procedure. The risk is higher for women with a retroverted (tipped or tilted) uterus who are given a transcervical CVS (about 5 in 100). For this reason, a transabdominal CVS (through the abdominal wall) is usually advised for these women. A consultation with a genetic counselor can help you analyze the positives and negatives and decide whether a CVS is right for you.

Fetal Monitoring

A fetal heart monitor measures the fetal heart rate (or FHR). A baseline (or average) fetal heart rate of 120–160 beats per minute (bpm) is considered normal. During your routine prenatal exams, a handheld monitor is used to quickly listen to the fetal heart rate. If you need to be monitored for a longer period of time, belts are used to keep the monitors in place for a period of about twenty minutes. When being monitored, your health care provider will look for fetal heart rate accelerations, which correspond to your baby's movement and are a sign of fetal well-being. Reasons to have the prolonged monitoring include going past your due date, IUGR, GDM, and other medical conditions.

Common Concerns: Heartburn and Hemorrhoids

Sometime in the second trimester, you may begin to experience heartburn, a burning feeling in your chest or throat. This feeling is due to stomach acid moving up into your esophagus. It's not uncommon in pregnancy and is due to your uterus crowding your stomach. Hormonal changes also have an effect by making muscles in your digestive tract remain relaxed rather than tightening to block acid movement out of the stomach.

There are some ways to reduce heartburn:

- Stay away from alcohol and caffeinated drinks; these can relax the valve between the stomach and the esophagus and exacerbate heartburn.
- Keep a food log to determine your heartburn triggers; many women find it helps to avoid greasy or spicy foods.
- Eat smaller, more frequent meals instead of three large ones.
- Don't eat just before you go to bed or lie down to rest.
- Rest your head on a few extra pillows in bed to assist gravity in easing heartburn while you sleep.

If heartburn symptoms won't relent, there are several over-the-counter antacids and medications available considered safe to use in pregnancy. Speak with your doctor to find the one right for you.

Being a vegan may help you avoid symptoms of another common condition, hemorrhoids. Hemorrhoids are swollen, inflamed veins around the anus or lower rectum. They can become itchy, painful, and perhaps even protrude from the anus. These swollen veins are caused by increased pressure from your growing uterus on the rectal veins coupled with pregnancy hormones that can cause veins to dilate and swell. When you strain to have a bowel movement or have a hard bowel movement, the hemorrhoid's fragile surface can be damaged and it can bleed. Vegan diets are typically high in fiber. This high fiber diet, along with exercise and plenty of water, can help you avoid constipation and straining with bowel movements that may aggravate hemorrhoids. If you do have painful hemorrhoids, try easing the pain with an ice pack, a soak in a warm tub, wipes with witch hazel pads, or a topical prescription cream as recommended by your doctor.

CHAPTER 14

The Third Trimester

It's the home stretch, the big countdown—the third trimester. You've made a lot of decisions so far, and there are even more to be made in the next few months. You'll be getting ready for labor and delivery as you sort through your options for childbirth classes and assemble a birth plan. You may feel some Braxton-Hicks contractions (discussed in an upcoming section in this chapter) as your body starts prepping for the hard work of labor. Consider them a dress rehearsal for the big event.

Your Body This Trimester

You're likely feeling perpetually stuffed and slightly out of breath as your uterus relocates all your internal organs. The relief and energy felt in the second trimester can start to fade now. Just remember, you're almost there!

At the beginning of this trimester, the top of the fundus (uterus) is halfway between your bellybutton and your breastbone, displacing your stomach, intestines, and diaphragm. It's increasingly easy to get winded as your little one pushes up into your diaphragm. Take it slow, breathe deeply, and practice good posture. To ease breathing while you sleep, pile on a few extra pillows or use a foam bed wedge to elevate your head.

Not only are your breasts heavier, but they are more glandular and getting ready to feed your baby. In this last trimester, your nipples may begin to leak colostrum, which is the yellowish, nutrient-rich fluid that precedes real breast milk. You may find the leaking more apparent when you're sexually aroused. To reduce backaches and breast tenderness, make sure you wear a well-fitting bra (even to bed if it helps). If you are planning on breastfeeding, you might want to consider buying some supportive nursing bras now that can take you through the rest of pregnancy and right into the postpartum period.

FACT

If you're picking up nursing bras, be sure to test drive the clasps for easy access. Try to unfasten and slip the nursing flaps down with one hand. This may seem unimportant now, but when you're in a crowded shopping mall trying to discreetly put baby to breast single handedly, you'll be thankful you had the foresight.

As baby settles firmly on your bladder, bathroom stops step up once again. You may even experience some stress incontinence, which is minor dribbling or leakage of urine when you sneeze, cough, laugh, or make other sudden movements. This will clear up postpartum. In the meantime, keep doing your Kegels (see Chapter 13), don't hold it in, and wear a pantyliner.

Braxton-Hicks Contractions

This trimester, your body is warming up for labor and you may start to experience Braxton-Hicks contractions. These painless and irregular contractions feel as if your uterus is making a fist and then gradually relaxing. If your little one is fairly active, you might think that he is stretching himself sideways at first. A quick check of your belly will reveal a visible tightening.

Braxton-Hicks can begin as early as week 20 and continue right up until your due date, although these contractions are more commonly felt in the final month of pregnancy. Some first time moms-to-be are afraid they won't be able to tell the difference between Braxton-Hicks and actual labor contractions. As any woman who has been through labor can attest, when the real thing comes, you'll know it. Rule of thumb: If it hurts, it's labor.

QUESTION

What if I don't get to the hospital in time?
The average labor lasts twelve to fourteen hours, plenty of time to get to the hospital. To avoid any unforeseen delays, work out a route in advance, keep your gas tank full, and have cash on hand for a cab in case your car conks out with the first contraction.

If your contractions suddenly seem to be coming at regular intervals and they start to cause you pain or discomfort, they could be the real thing. Lie down on your left side for about a half hour with a clock or watch on hand and time the contractions from the beginning of one to the beginning of the next. If the interludes are more or less regular, call your health care provider. And if contractions of any type are accompanied by blood or amniotic fluid leakage, contact your practitioner immediately.

Your Body—Changes in the Last Month

Engagement (or lightening), the process of the baby dropping down into the pelvic cavity in preparation for delivery, can occur any time now. In some women, particularly those who have given birth before, it may not happen until labor starts.

Your cervix is ripening (softening) in preparation for baby's passage. As it effaces (thins) and dilates (opens), the soft plug of mucus keeping it sealed tight may be dislodged. This mass, which has the appealing name of *mucous plug*, may be tinged red or pink.

If the baby has dropped, you could be running to the bathroom more than ever. She also may be sending shockwaves through your pelvis as she settles further down onto the pelvic floor. On the up side, you can finally breathe as she pulls away from your lungs and diaphragm. Braxton-Hicks contractions can be more frequent this month as you draw nearer to delivery. You're close enough to be on the lookout for the real thing, however. How will you recognize them?

Real contractions will:

- Be felt in the back and possibly radiate around to the abdomen.
- *Not* subside when you move around or change positions.
- Increase in intensity as time passes.
- Come at roughly regular intervals (early on, this can be from twenty to forty-five minutes apart).
- Increase in intensity with activity like walking.

Other signs that labor is on its way include amniotic fluid that leaks in either a gush or a trickle (your "water breaking"), sudden diarrhea, and the appearance of the mucous plug. Keep in mind, however, that for many women, the bag of waters does not break until active labor sets in.

At the Doctor

This trimester, your visits to the doctor might start to step up to twice monthly, with weekly visits in the last month. Your provider will probably want to know whether you've been experiencing any Braxton-Hicks contractions, and he will cover the warning signs of preterm labor and what you should do if you experience them.

Sometime in your eighth month, your practitioner will check the position of your baby to determine whether she has turned head down in preparation for birth. You may learn that your baby is in breech position (bottom or foot first).

Don't panic. Your fickle fetus is likely to change position again in the next few weeks. If she doesn't, your practitioner may try to turn the baby closer to term.

ALERT

Amniotic fluid is clear to straw-colored and has a faintly sweet smell. Less commonly, it may be tinged green or brown. If you think you're leaking amniotic fluid, no matter how small the amount, contact your care provider. If your membranes have ruptured, you risk infection if you don't deliver soon.

In the last month, unless you are scheduled for a planned cesarean, your provider will probably perform an internal exam with each visit to check your cervix for changes that indicate approaching labor. He'll also be taking note of any descent or dropping of the baby toward the pelvis. Although you may start effacing and dilating now, it's still anyone's guess as to when labor will begin, and it could be a few more weeks yet.

On Your Mind

As labor looms closer, your thoughts turn to the task at hand. Going into labor and delivery with as much knowledge of the process as possible can make the difference between a positive childbirth experience and a frustrating one.

Am I Up to the Task of Labor?

Women have been doing this since the beginning of time and under much more difficult circumstances. Yes, in most cases labor will be hard work, but if you prepare yourself by learning what to expect, you will be ready to face whatever comes your way. You'll also find that your spouse or labor partner and coach will be a huge asset in helping you through childbirth.

Am I Up to the Task of Motherhood?

Great mommies are made, not born. Although some aspects of mothering will seem to come to you instinctively, practice and trial and error will make up the better part of your parenting education. Use the tools around you—your pediatrician, other mothers, and research and reading—to build and sharpen your skills. In the final analysis, listen to your inner voice in the application of what you learn.

Nesting

Nesting is that overwhelming urge to prepare a safe haven for your little one and assure yourself that all his needs and wants will be adequately met. You may be trying to furnish a nursery and clean the house—both instinctive reactions to the upcoming arrival.

Keep in mind that during the first few weeks home, keeping baby within arm's length will improve your rest and peace of mind. A bassinet can make her feel safer and more secure than in the open space of a crib, after spending nine months in close quarters. And you can roll a bassinet right next to your bed to give those 4 A.M. feedings with ease.

ESSENTIAL

Some baby essentials you should have on hand prior to his arrival: diapers, wipes, alcohol swabs (for his umbilical cord), vegan baby shampoo and soap, vegan diaper-rash ointment, waterproof pads, bottles, a thermometer, and a fever-reducing product (Tylenol) recommended by your pediatrician.

Don't go crazy buying supersized cases of baby supplies; buy small so you can sample. Once you've decided what works best for you and baby, you can stock up. Now is the time to start thinking about whether you want to go cloth or disposable with diapers. If you're thinking green, cloth diapers have the advantage of not ending up in a landfill, although they do require additional fossil fuels and water resources to wash and transport (if you use a service). Call local diaper services to get estimates and a rundown of what's included. You can wash diapers at home, of course, but be sure you have the time to be doing laundry daily. If your baby has sensitive skin, you might find cloth less irritating. Like most things in parenting, it's trial and error—have a supply of both and see how each works for you.

Setting Up a Vegan Nursery

Most baby supplies, from diaper-rash cream to baby shampoo, are available in vegan versions. Check a well-stocked natural foods store or co-op or look for online vegan supply companies. See Appendix A for a list of companies. You may want to start by buying small sizes to see which brands you prefer. Check with other parents on vegetarian parent electronic mail lists to see if there are brands that other parents recommend.

On Your Mind—The Last Month

You are so ready to have this baby. Nothing fits, not even your shoes. You can't sleep for more than a few hours at a time. You look toward your due date like a long distance runner approaching the end of a marathon. As you waddle toward the finish line, enjoy these final sensations of your child moving inside of you—the funny little hiccups, the elbow and knee bumps parading across your belly, and the subtle nudges that remind you you're not alone even if no one else is around. Relish these final days of exhilaration and anticipation—they are unique.

First-time moms may find themselves overwhelmed with anxiety now that birth is so near. Take a deep breath, go over what you learned in childbirth class, and talk with your partner or labor coach about ways to get past the anxious feelings. It's perfectly natural to be fearful of the unknown, but don't let fear wrest control of your labor from you.

Even if you have been through pregnancy already, you might still be anxious about baby's arrival. Perhaps you're following a different kind of labor and birth plan or you're concerned about how your other child will react to his new sibling. Again, talk it out with your partner, ask your provider any questions that are still on your mind about labor and delivery, and remember that you've been through this once and you'll make it through again.

Childbirth Classes

Most childbirth seminars available through hospitals and birthing centers are called *prepared childbirth classes*. Taking place in a classroom setting and using lectures, audiovisuals, and floor exercises to get you ready for labor and delivery, prepared childbirth classes usually focus on one, two, or more birth philosophies. They can vary in length from several months of Saturdays to a one-day seminar. While hospital policy will dictate a lot of what's covered, you can expect to get a guided tour of the facility, learn what goes on in labor and delivery, and find out some basics of caring for a new baby. Your husband, partner, or labor coach will learn more about their role in the process. You'll get all sorts of brochures, handouts, and forms that you can read at home. Perhaps the most important facet of childbirth class (and certainly the one that most first-time moms pay the closest attention to) is the information it provides on managing labor and delivery discomforts. In addition to an overview of anesthesia and pain medication options, childbirth educators draw on one or more childbirth philosophies to teach coping methods.

To find out about what's available, call your hospital or birthing center and ask for schedules and descriptions of upcoming classes. Once you get a feel for what is offered, call with follow-up questions about instructor credentials and training, methods taught, class size, curriculum, and costs. You might also ask if there are couples who have taken the course that you can contact as references.

ESSENTIAL

If you've had a previous cesarean section, ask about a VBAC class, which provides couples with information on the benefits, risks, and statistics surrounding vaginal births following a cesarean section. They are usually recommended as a supplement to, rather than a replacement for, a prepared childbirth class.

Even if you don't choose a childbirth class sponsored by the facility where you'll be giving birth, you should try to arrange a tour. Getting your bearings ahead of time will save you valuable time and frustration when the big day arrives. You'll also have less anxiety if you know what to expect of the labor and birthing rooms.

New sibling classes can be a huge boon for families with other children. Typically divided by age group so information can be communicated at an appropriate level, these classes put an emphasis on how things at home are changing, how the family will adjust after baby is born, and what the children are feeling about these developments. A sibling class can help your child feel more involved in, and consequently more accepting of, your family's growth.

Writing Your Birth Plan

Are you looking forward to a completely chemical-free birth or are you already exploring your painkilling options? Do you want only your partner in attendance or would you like additional support? Your birth plan is your chance to let everyone involved know what you want the experience to be. Whatever your idea of perfect labor and delivery is, make sure the direction of your birth plan is driven by the needs of your partner and you and not by the expectations of others. Remember, of course, that plans can change as conditions change during labor and delivery. Appendix B in the back of this book includes a checklist you can use for guidance in creating your birth plan. Also take a look at the next chapter, which provides more information about labor and delivery.

Developing a birth plan can ease your anxieties and serve as a springboard for discussions with your partner. Because the plan can tread on some sensitive and controversial medical territory, it's important that your provider be included in the process.

Working with Your Provider

Once you and your partner have your birth plan together, you should present it to your provider for his comments and questions. Communicating your wishes and being receptive to feedback can make the difference between a birth plan that works and one that doesn't.

Consider the plan you initially take to your provider a first draft. Be willing to really listen to any suggestions or issues your provider has and make an effort to work toward a resolution together. Also, try to keep your expectations grounded in reality and not overly restrictive. After your discussion, you can incorporate your provider's input into your final plan.

While covering all your bases is important, you simply can't control every possible aspect of what does or doesn't occur during labor and delivery. Medical emergencies do happen, which is why you have signed on a practitioner to begin with. You need to trust your provider to follow the spirit of your birth plan while making adjustments for your health and that of your baby. Establishing a good communicative relationship is the best way to ensure this.

Your doctor will warn you up front that unforeseen circumstances will mean a deviation from your birth plan. Sometimes women feel as if they have failed if matters do not go precisely according to their concept of *the ideal birth,* which is certainly not realistic. The best way to avoid disappointment is to build alternative scenarios into your birth plan regarding interventions that might be required. For example, if you really don't want an episiotomy, you should indicate that in your birth plan and suggest perineal massage with vitamin E oil or another lubricant, warm compresses, or another acceptable alternative. But be prepared to work with your doctor during labor if your alternative plan just doesn't do the trick.

Some vegans will wonder if medications and supplies used in their treatment are vegan. The Vegan Society in the U.K. maintains a listing of animal-free medications at *www.vegansociety.com/healthcare/gps/animal-free-medications-list.aspx.* This list is not comprehensive and may not include medications available in the United States. You can certainly ask your doctor if vegan alternatives are available for commonly used medications (if the medication is supplied in a gelatin-based capsule, it may also be available as a liquid or tablet). You can also discuss your preference for vegan medications and supplies. However, in many cases practitioners simply don't know if medications are vegan or not. Try to do your best, keep in mind that your health and the well-being of your baby are very important, and that your dietary choices are already promoting a more humane world.

Gearing Up for the Big Event

Since baby's timetable is somewhat unpredictable, start getting your affairs in order at the beginning of the ninth month. Cover all personal, professional, and family bases to ensure a smooth transition from home to hospital and back home again. For example, double check with your provider that a copy of your birth plan has been put into your chart, and verify any changes you might have made to the plan since your first review together.

Being Vegan in the Hospital

Most hospitals, sad to say, don't routinely serve vegan meals. If you'd prefer not to pick at a salad and maybe some steamed vegetables during your stay, some planning ahead of time is key. Start by reminding your doctor that you are vegan so that a vegan diet order can be placed on your chart. Contact the dietary department at the hospital prior to your due date, describe your diet, and ask how they will meet your needs. Ask about bringing some of your own food, especially basics like soymilk. Can your partner supply vegan takeout for a post-delivery celebratory meal? Be sure to find out who to contact and how to contact them should anything go wrong once you're in the hospital.

Pack Your Bag

You'll probably pack and unpack your bag a half dozen times this month making sure you have everything you could possibly need. Don't go crazy with work or entertainment equipment—you'll be too busy with labor, delivery, and meeting and caring for your child.

Essentials you should have:

❑ **Pain-relief tools and music for labor.** Things like massage balls, a picture for focusing on through contractions, a water bottle. Check with your hospital or birthing center to see whether a small portable stereo is acceptable. If not, bring personal headphones.

❑ **Snacks for the coach.** Make sure it's something that won't turn your stomach during labor.

❑ **A camera.** For capturing baby's arrival (or the moments shortly thereafter). Don't forget batteries and an extra memory card!

❑ **Stopwatch or watch with a second hand.** For timing contractions.

❑ **Clothes for you.** Include several nightgowns with button or snap fronts if you're going to nurse, a bathrobe, extra underwear, socks and/

or slippers for those cold floors, and something loose and comfortable to wear to go home. And be sure to bring glasses or contacts if you need them.

❏ **Sanitary pads.** The hospital will provide you with some, but extras are good to have on hand.

❏ **Phone numbers.** Bring names and numbers of the folks you'll want to call immediately.

❏ **Something for siblings.** A big sister/brother gift and their photo on the newborn's bassinet can make their introduction smoother.

❏ **Toiletries and shower supplies.** Bring your chosen brand of vegan toothpaste, shampoo, and other basics along with a toothbrush.

❏ **A going-home outfit for baby.** Pack a set of newborn clothes and a baby blanket. Let your partner bring the car seat on discharge day.

If you're breastfeeding, you might also pack:
❏ **Nursing bras.** If you don't have any yet, a bra with a front fastener will work well as a stand-in for now.

❏ **A box of nursing pads.** For when your milk comes in.

❏ **Vitamin E oil or vegan ointment.** For sore or cracked nipples.

Recruit Help Now!

Now is the time to take friends, family, and neighbors up on their offers of assistance. If they ask whether they can help, say yes! Make a list and schedule assignments. Give friends who are good in the kitchen ideas for easy vegan meals they can prepare for you. If you have other children, make sure their schedules are covered.

Feel like you need some live-in help to get you through the first week or so? Ask a mommy expert, maybe your own mom, to come for a visit. Sound out the idea with your mate—they may feel this is a special family time, but might reconsider if they hear your reasons. Just make sure your guest isn't someone who will add to your stress.

Finalize Maternity-Leave Plans

If you're working right up until your due date, start clearing the decks early in the month. Make sure coworkers and managers are regularly apprised of where outstanding projects stand, and try to treat every day as if it might be your last before you leave. The more you enable matters to flow smoothly in your absence, the less likely you are to get calls at home.

Talk with your supervisor about communication during your absence. If you want to remain incommunicado (and you have every right to do so), make your feelings known. You might limit any contact you do agree to, such as e-mails only or phone calls only in a certain window of time each day. Remember, this is your time off both to recuperate and to get to know your child.

Hurry Up and Wait (When Baby Is Late)

You've finally reached that magic EDD and...nothing. Don't be too depressed. Instead, try to stay busy, and if you feel up to it, get out and about. Unless you have a precise twenty-eight-day cycle and are positive of the exact day that sperm met egg, gestational dating can be fuzzy at best. If you are a week or more past the EDD, your provider will order additional tests that will give her a better picture of whether or not baby is ready to arrive.

Babies who stay in the womb 42 weeks or longer are considered post-date. Postdate pregnancies can develop *macrosomia*, or large body size (8 pounds, 13 ounces or more) that could make it difficult to pass through the birth canal. A postdate fetus may also pass meconium, which, if released into the amniotic fluid, has the potential to cause lung problems after birth. Postdate pregnancies are also associated with an increased risk of still-birth and placental insufficiency (when the placenta can no longer provide enough oxygen and nutrients to the baby). That's why regular assessment of a postdate pregnancy is extremely important.

CHAPTER 15

Labor and Delivery

Even if you've read up on labor and delivery, took copious notes in every session of childbirth class, and questioned your friends on their birth experiences, you'll still find your labor is different in some way from that of others. Because every woman's labor is unique (as is each birth), comparisons of length, progress, and pain perception can be inaccurate and even discouraging. Follow your own path and you'll do fine.

Get Ready: Baby and Your Body in Labor

Labor is hard work (don't let anyone tell you otherwise), but it's also the most rewarding work you'll ever do.

Contractions

The first signal of labor is contractions—the tightening and release of your uterus that helps propel your baby down the birth canal. These contractions differ from the Braxton-Hicks ones you've possibly had in that they occur at regular intervals, are painful, and are slowly but surely opening the door (that is, cervix) for baby's exit.

ESSENTIAL

If you don't want to be bound to your bed during labor, find out whether your birth facility has fetal monitors that use telemetry. These wireless monitors strap on like a regular external device so that you don't have to remain plugged into anything. There are even telemetry units that are waterproof, if you plan on easing labor pains with hydrotherapy.

When contractions start, call your practitioner to let her know labor has started and how far apart contractions are. Remember, contractions are timed from the beginning of one to the start of the next. Your provider will let you know at what point you should head for the hospital or birthing center.

Prep

When you do arrive at your birthing center or hospital, the nursing staff will prep (or prepare) you for labor and delivery. You'll start by changing into your hospital gown or nightgown from home. Depending on your facility's policy, you could be getting a partial shave of your perineal area or, less commonly, a full shave of both your abdominal and pubic area.

Your nurse may insert a needle with a heparin lock and secure it with surgical tape. If intravenous (IV) medication is suddenly needed during labor, it can be easily hooked up. Other hospitals will hook you up to an IV line as a matter of course and administer a glucose solution to keep you hydrated. Other medications can be added to the line as necessary. You may be hooked up to fetal and uterine monitors that will allow you and your coach to see when a contraction is coming and, more important, when it seems to be almost over. It will also pick up fetal heart sounds and alert your medical team to any stress the baby may be experiencing. An internal monitor might be used if you are considered to be at high risk. (For more on fetal monitoring, turn back to Chapter 13.)

Get Set: Pain-Relief Options

In early labor when contractions are getting intense but are still not close enough to leave for the hospital, there are a few ways you can ease the pain.

Nonmedical Solutions

Experiment with different positions, such as on all fours, against a wall, and leaning against someone or something while bent forward at the waist.

Back labor, which occurs when baby's face is toward your abdomen rather than toward your spine, can cause severe lower back pain. Ask your partner to try massage or a warm water bottle to ease contractions. The soothing jets of a whirlpool tub can do wonders, if you have one. If your water has broken, however, never take a soak without approval from your provider.

Keep positive, supportive people around you. Let your coach be your buffer and clear out any distractions. Try to remain focused on riding through and past the contraction. Fix your eyes on something that relaxes you and practice the breathing exercises you learned in childbirth class to keep the oxygen and blood flowing. Don't hyperventilate. Talk or groan through the peak of the contraction if it helps. Letting go in between contractions can help ease your mind and body and loosen you up for impending delivery. Use the relaxation exercises that you learned in childbirth class.

Pharmaceutical Options

Once you arrive at the hospital, you will have analgesics and anesthetics available for pain relief, if you choose to use them.

Analgesics

Analgesics deaden the pain by depressing your nervous system. They make you sleepy and help you rest between contractions. The analgesics Demerol (meperidine), Stadol (butorphanol), Nubain (nalbuphine), and Sublimaze (fentanyl) are commonly used in labor. Although these medications can cross the placenta, when they are properly administered in the appropriate dosages they should not cause baby any serious side effects.

Local Anesthesia

Local anesthesia, also called *regional anesthesia*, numbs only a specific portion of the body, and leaves you awake and alert. The most commonly used local anesthesia is probably the lumbar epidural. Injected into the space between two vertebrae of your lower back (the epidural space), this type of anesthesia is administered when you are well into labor, and will temporarily numb the nerves all the way from your bellybutton to your knees. An epidural takes twenty minutes to start working, and can lower your blood pressure. For this reason, you'll be put on the fetal monitor and hooked up to an IV fluid drip if you're given an epidural. The numbness will take several hours to wear off and may restrict your movements during the birth, but an epidural can be a great pain-management tool.

FACT

A spinal block is similar to an epidural in that it's administered in the lower back. However, a spinal is delivered directly into your lower spine, not into the spaces between your vertebrae as in an epidural. Used right at delivery only or during a C-section, the spinal will numb you all the way from your rib cage down.

Women who want the pain-relief benefits of an epidural but also to retain the ability to move around during labor are candidates for a low-dose combination spinal epidural, sometimes referred to as a walking epidural. A walking epidural is usually faster acting than a conventional epidural and allows you to retain enough sensation to move and walk, which can speed the labor process.

General Anesthesia

General anesthesia is rarely used in labor and delivery, except in cases of an emergency cesarean section when there isn't adequate time to prep the patient with a local anesthetic. It brings about a complete loss of consciousness. Newborns arriving under the influence of a general anesthesia can be drowsy and slow to respond.

Go! Labor in Three Acts

Labor is a series of three distinct stages, aptly called first, second, and third stages. For most women, the longest span is the first stage, which lasts from the earliest signs of labor right through baby's descent into the birth canal in preparation for stage two—pushing. Stage three consists of delivering the placenta, which mothers usually feel is a cakewalk after all the hard work involved in baby's arrival.

First Stage

The first stage of labor begins with early labor and ends with active labor. Your provider probably uses the term *transition* (or *descent*) to refer to the end of the first stage of labor.

ESSENTIAL

If your birthing center or hospital has whirlpool tubs or showers available for laboring moms, you might find the pulsating water welcome relief for getting through contractions. This pain-relief method (called *hydrotherapy*) is not the same as a water birth, in which a baby is actually born submerged in a pool of water.

During the early phase the cervix effaces (thins) and dilates (opens). This process may have started several weeks ago. Now your cervix will dilate to 4–5 centimeters. Contractions will arrive every 15–20 minutes and last 60–90 seconds. Try to stay up and moving through contractions as much as you can to let gravity help your baby descend. Use the breathing and relaxation techniques you picked up in childbirth class to get you through these first few hours. Then leave for the hospital and the next phase—active labor.

In active labor, your contractions are coming closer together regularly, perhaps 3–5 minutes apart, and they can be intense, lasting 45–60 seconds. These strong contractions are dilating your cervix from about 4–5 centimeters to around 8.

Don't feel inadequate or guilty about asking for pain medication at any point if you want it. Pain medication is a tool, just like your breathing exercises. Wisely used, it can result in a better birth experience for both you and your child.

Once your cervix reaches 8 centimeters and contractions start coming one on top of the other to get you to full dilation, the end of the first stage has arrived. Because of the frequency of contractions and the overwhelming urge to push, this is the most difficult part of labor. Fortunately, it culminates in your child's delivery, once you bridge those final 2 centimeters to become fully dilated.

As you begin to transition from first- to second-stage labor:

- You could be nauseous and may even vomit.
- You have chills or sweats, and your muscles twitch.
- Your back *really, really* hurts.
- Contractions are just minutes apart, if even that.
- There is pressure in your rectum from the baby.
- You are absolutely exhausted.
- You may feel like pushing even though your cervix is not yet fully dilated.

Although every fiber of your body is probably screaming, "PUSH!" you need to hold back just a few moments more. Your cervix is almost but not quite open far enough for baby's safe passage. Take quick, shallow breaths and resist the urge to push until your doctor or midwife gives the go ahead.

Second Stage or PUSH!

Your cervix has made it to 10 centimeters, and you are finally allowed to push. This second stage can last anywhere from a few minutes (with second or subsequent babies) to several hours. Your contractions will still arrive regularly, but they aren't quite as close together—a welcome relief. Pushing is very hard work, but the sensations may change from the intense gripping you've experienced to more of a stinging or burning sensation.

ESSENTIAL

If possible, try to find a pushing position that makes you feel comfortable and in control. Use gravity to your advantage by kneeling, squatting, or sitting up with your legs and knees spread far apart. Stirrups are likely available, but don't feel forced into using them if they don't work for you.

Your birth attendant and/or coach will let you know when the peak of the contraction occurs, the optimum time for pushing effectively. Use whatever it takes to push effectively. If that means moaning, grunting, and emitting other primal sounds that make your prenatal snoring sound like a lullaby by comparison, go for it. The people attending your birth have probably heard just about everything. Don't be embarrassed, because the noise won't even faze them.

You may be asked to stop pushing momentarily as the baby's head is ready to emerge, in order to prevent perineal tearing. Panting can help you suppress the urge. The obstetrician or midwife may decide on an episiotomy if your skin doesn't appear willing to stretch another millimeter or she may attempt perineal massage.

Finally, the head slides face down past the perineum and is eased out carefully to prevent injury to the baby. The attendant may wipe the eyes, nose, and mouth and suction any mucus or fluid from her upper respiratory tract. It's all downhill, from here as the rest of the body slides out.

As your baby leaves the quiet, dim warmth of the womb, his respiratory reflexes kick in and the newborn lungs fill with air for the first time. He'll probably test out those lungs with a full-fledged wail. Your doctor will place the baby on your stomach for introductions, usually with the umbilical cord still attached.

Third Stage or You Aren't Done Yet!

The third stage of labor is the delivery of the placenta. The entire placenta must be expelled to prevent bleeding and infection complications later on. Contractions will continue, and your doctor may press down on your abdomen and massage your uterus or tug gently on the end of the umbilical cord hanging from your vagina. You might also be injected with the hormone Pitocin (oxytocin) to step up your contractions and expel the placenta. Once the placenta is out, any stitches you require to repair tearing or episiotomy incisions will be put in. A local anesthetic will be injected to deaden the area if you aren't still anesthetized from an epidural.

Cesarean Section

A cesarean birth will be scheduled for you if you have a breech baby or other complications or conditions that indicate the need for such. It may also be performed in emergency situations in which the fetus is in distress. A cesarean is major abdominal surgery and carries with it all the risks of infection and complication that any surgical procedure does. On the positive side, with a planned C-section, the date your physician schedules the procedure is your due date, and no contractions are necessary unless you begin to labor before that time.

In Advance of the Surgery

If you have any advance warning about your C-section, you'll probably be offered an epidural or spinal rather than general anesthesia. Before the procedure begins, you'll be prepped. A nurse may shave the area of the incision, and your arm will be hooked up to an intravenous line to receive fluids as well as pain medication. You may also be asked to drink an antacid solution called *sodium citrate* to neutralize your stomach acid.

Before the procedure begins, you will have a catheter inserted into your bladder. The anesthetic block will give you little control over the muscles that control urine flow, so the catheter will do the work for you both during and after the procedure. Catheter insertion can be uncomfortable, so ask that it be inserted after you've received your anesthetic block (which will likely be in the operating room).

In the Operating Room

Once you're prepped, you will be wheeled to the operating room. In the operating room, the anesthesiologist will place the epidural or spinal block into your back. You'll then be asked to lie flat on your back with your arms straight out to the sides. A curtain just a few feet high will be positioned at your chest to keep the surgical field (the area where all the action is) sterile. This will also block your view of the procedure, so if you're determined to see baby the moment she emerges, you will want to ask for an appropriately placed mirror as early as possible.

Your arms may be loosely fastened down with Velcro straps. This is to prevent any accidental movements that could breech the sterility of the surgical field.

The most uncomfortable part of the C-section procedure is arguably the flat-on-your-back part. It's quite possible you will get nauseous as your heavy uterus compresses your vena cava and starts to lower your blood pressure. In addition, the anesthetic itself may cause your blood pressure to fall. Although the anesthesiologist will administer medication to control this drop (called *hypotension*), you may get sick to your stomach. The discomfort is compounded by the fact that you will have to vomit lying down with your head turned to the side. This is where a well-placed mate, tray in hand, is indispensable. Hang in there and remember this part will likely be short lived.

The obstetrician will make an incision, and the baby's head, perfectly round because she hasn't done battle with the birth canal, will be lifted out first and her mouth and nose suctioned. As your doctor helps your baby out of the incision, you'll feel a strange pulling sensation. Once the cord is cut, you'll be able to finally see your baby, albeit briefly, before he is taken for assessment and a quick cleanup by the nursing staff. In some cases the pediatric team will be in the operating room to assess the baby immediately. Your incision will be stitched closed, and you'll be wheeled off to the recovery room where your little one will meet up with you once again. The entire surgical procedure will only take about thirty to forty-five minutes.

Emergency C-Section

If your C-section is performed under emergency circumstances, events could move quickly and you'll have fewer options. You could also be given a general anesthetic that will make you unconscious. Most partners are asked to step outside once general anesthesia has been administered, but you might want to talk to your doctor about special circumstances during childbirth.

Induction

In cases where you are definitely 41 weeks or further along and it seems your child is perfectly content to spend his infancy in your womb, your practitioner may recommend induction. Inducing labor involves both helping the cervix ripen for baby's passage and stimulating uterine contractions; both are important for a successful labor and delivery.

Your provider may use one of several methods to facilitate cervical ripening, including membrane stripping and amniotomy (manual breaking of the membranes or bag of waters). Stripping (or sweeping) of the membranes is simply the separation of the amniotic membrane from the wall of the cervix. Your provider will insert her finger in the cervix and gently sweep it between the amniotic membrane and the uterine wall.

If she opts for amniotomy, she'll use an instrument with a small blunt hook on the end to break through the amniotic sac. With the latter method, if labor does not start on its own within twenty-four hours, scheduled induction may be necessary because of the risk of infection for the baby.

Because a scheduled induction is more successful when the cervix is prepared for the experience, your practitioner may recommend an application of prostaglandin to your cervix the day prior or in the hospital. The prostaglandin helps ripen the cervix for labor and delivery. In some cases it can be used alone as an inducing agent. The prostaglandin can take the form of a gel or tablet and can be inserted into the vagina. On some occasions, the tablet is given orally. The baby's heart rate is assessed with a fetal monitor after the prostaglandin is given and during labor. More than one application may be ordered.

Manual dilators and Foley catheters can also be used for cervical ripening, as an alternative to the use of drugs. The type of cervical ripening method used depends on your personal preference, your medical history, and the cervical exam.

Pitocin, a synthetic formulation of the hormone oxytocin that stimulates uterine contractions, may be prescribed as an inducing agent. The hormone is given intravenously, and you will be hooked up to a fetal monitor to monitor your baby's progress.

According to the CDC, more than one in five births were induced in 2005. Researchers attribute the increase to earlier prenatal care, wider availability of induction agents, and nonmedical reasons such as convenience for the patient or doctor. Because induction can cause intense contractions and result in a longer labor, its use should always be carefully considered.

After the Birth

The pinnacle of nine months of physical chaos and emotional oscillation, of queasy stomach, aches, pains, and hair-trigger laughter and tears has arrived. Your baby is here, placed skin to skin to feel his mother's outside warmth for the very first time.

Meeting Baby

A thousand different feelings and emotions, from utter exhaustion to indescribable joy, will flood you as you look down at that little scrunched face, still adjusting to his new waterless environment. Wrapped in a blanket with a little stocking cap to keep his head warm, he looks so perfect yet so vulnerable.

If you're planning on breastfeeding, you can nurse him while you get acquainted, even in the recovery room if you've had a C-section. It's awe-inspiring how he knows just what to do, instinctively rooting for your breast with his eyes barely open and then latching on. Spend as long as you want getting familiar, and let your partner share in the bonding, too. This is a precious time for your new family.

Baby's First Doctor's Visit

Your baby will have some initial tests and treatments to ensure a healthy welcome into the world. The first is an Apgar test. Created by noted pediatrician Dr. Virginia Apgar, the Apgar measures Appearance (skin color), Pulse, Grimace (reflexes), Activity, and Respiration. The Apgar is given just one minute after birth and again five minutes after that. The attendant will assign a score of 0 to 2 for each category and add the numbers together for the total Apgar. An average score is 7–10.

After the Apgar, your newborn will be measured, weighed, and have prints taken of her feet and fingers. Silver nitrate or antibiotic eye drops or ointment may be put in her eyes to prevent infection from anything she encountered in the birth canal. She'll also receive a vitamin K injection to prevent bleeding problems; a heel-stick blood draw to test for PKU and hypothyroidism; and in some hospitals a hepatitis B vaccine. Further tests may be administered if you have a chronic illness or have experienced complications during pregnancy.

Taking Care of Mom

After the birth, you'll have some assistance cleaning up and will be given a good supply of super-absorbent sanitary pads. You'll also be provided with a peribottle, a plastic squirt bottle used to cleanse and soothe your perineal area with warm water each time you use the bathroom.

ALERT

If bleeding is soaking more than a pad an hour, let your provider know. It could be a sign that a piece of placenta is still retained in your uterus. This condition usually requires surgical removal of the placental fragments, called *curettage*.

You'll be expelling lochia for up to six weeks following birth, whether you've had a vaginal birth or a C-section. Lochia—a mixture of blood, mucus, and tissue that comes from the implantation site of the placenta—will be quite heavy in the days immediately following the birth, so don't be alarmed.

If you've had a C-section, you'll spend some time in the recovery area before heading to your hospital room. Your incision will be checked regularly and pain medication will be administered as needed. The next day you'll be encouraged to walk as soon as possible to get your digestive tract active again, and you'll be asked about your gas and bathroom habits ad nauseum. The nursing staff is just trying to ensure that everything is returning to normal in gastrointestinal land.

Women who are given episiotomies will take sitz baths (also known as hip baths) to relieve pain, promote healing, and keep the area clean. A sitz bath is a small shallow tub of water, sometimes with medication added, that you sit in. Some mild pain relievers may also be prescribed to ease episiotomy pain.

If you are planning on breastfeeding, now is the perfect time to get your technique down. Your OB nurses will likely ask you how breastfeeding is progressing and can examine your latching technique to help you troubleshoot if breastfeeding isn't yet going smoothly. In some cases, there is even a lactation consultant available, and hospitals frequently offer breastfeeding classes to their new-mother inpatients. (For more on breastfeeding, see Chapter 16.)

Remember that even though it will take a few days for your breasts to start manufacturing milk, you are still providing your child with nutrient-rich colostrum, the prelude to breast milk. When your milk does *come in*, about the third day after delivery, your breasts can be quite swollen, hard, and sore. This engorgement will be relieved upon nursing. If you're going the bottle route, cold packs and supportive bras or binding can ease the discomfort. The tenderness of engorgement usually passes in two to three days and can be relieved by mild analgesics as prescribed by your doctor.

CHAPTER 16

Feeding Your Baby

Breastfeeding is part instinct, part practice, and a whole lot of persistence and patience. It's this last part that makes the difference between breast and bottle for many women, particularly in the first weeks of motherhood when even minor nursing difficulties can seem insurmountable. Stick with it, and get help and advice from other moms and from your health care providers. The good news is that breastfeeding usually becomes easier and more fulfilling over time. And in case you were wondering, breastfed babies of well-nourished vegan women grow and thrive.

Breast or Bottle?

Are you going to breastfeed or go the formula route? It's an issue over which many new moms feel intense pressure, and if you're still undecided, you've likely heard extensive opinions on both sides of the subject. Which is the right choice?

If you compare breast milk to formula strictly on a nutrient basis, few would disagree that the better choice is breast milk. Human milk is designed to meet the needs of human babies. But since the issue is also loaded with social, emotional, and personal considerations, the matter is seldom so black and white. In the end, breast or bottle is an individual choice.

Reasons for Breastfeeding

Breast milk is custom made to meet your baby's nutritional needs. It provides her with essential antibodies that can boost her immune system, leading to fewer colds, ear infections, and stomach upsets. Breastfed babies are also less likely to develop allergies and asthma, so if you have a significant family history of allergies, breastfeeding is recommended.

Breastfeeding gives your baby some significant life-long advantages. Breastfed babies have a lower risk of developing diabetes, heart disease, and childhood leukemia. They're also less likely to become overweight children and thereby less likely to have weight problems in adulthood. Breastfed infants have even been shown to have higher IQs and to do better in school through their high school years. Breastfeeding can also offer health benefits to you. Many women who breastfeed experience faster postpartum weight loss, especially if they breastfeed for at least six months. In addition, breastfeeding reduces your risk of developing diabetes and breast and ovarian cancer.

Breastfeeding is a low-maintenance feeding routine. Breast milk is always close at hand and never needs mixing, warming, or other preparation. You don't have to remember to pack sterilized bottles and nipples, formula, bottled water for mixing powdered formula, a can opener for opening premixed formula, and an ice pack if you've made the bottles in advance. If you're on a budget, breastfeeding is a big cost cutter. Aside from the high cost of formula itself, you can save on bottles, bags, cleaning gadgets, and other formula-feeding purchases. Of course, you'll be eating a bit more, but the cost of your extra food is low compared to the costs associated with formula feeding.

QUESTION

I'm going back to work soon. Should I even bother breastfeeding now?
Even a short period of breastfeeding can have big advantages for your baby. Many women do return to work and continue to nurse. Pumping breast milk or gradually reducing the number of feedings to nurse in the morning and the evening only (and supplement with formula) are options.

Nursing also gives you special one-on-one bonding time with baby. And as a breastfeeding mom, you're taking part in a tradition as old as motherhood itself and giving your child something no one else can. The experience is priceless.

Being Comfortable with Your Decision

If you have a medical condition that requires drug treatment, it's possible your medication can pass into breast milk and pose a risk to baby. This could be a reason to decide to bottle feed. There are other good reasons why breastfeeding is not a workable option for you. You are not an uncaring and self-absorbed mother if you choose to bottle feed.

Try to weigh the risks versus the benefits in your situation. All things being equal, women who are well supported at home, are healthy, and don't face an excessively demanding work schedule should consider giving breastfeeding a try, even if they feel a little awkward about it. Often the awkwardness evaporates with a little practice and through the bond forged with baby in nursing. And the health benefits gained by baby will last a lifetime.

On the other hand, if you're a single mom who works two jobs and is already stretched to the limit emotionally and physically, don't be pressured into breastfeeding by others because it is "the right thing to do." Excessive stress can do more damage than good, impairing your parenting skills, putting your health at risk, and straining the time the two of you do have together. Not every life situation is ideal for breastfeeding, even if you are capable of doing it. Make the decision that works best for your family.

Your Body and Breastfeeding

As soon as you can hold baby, you can breastfeed him. In the first few days following birth, your breasts will produce a clear to yellow sticky substance called *colostrum*. Colostrum contains antibodies that help strengthen the infant immune system. It is also important for getting baby's digestion off on the right track. The low-carbohydrate, high-protein concoction is easily digestible in these early days and helps establish intestinal flora, a beneficial bacteria, in baby's gastrointestinal tract. It also encourages the passing of meconium, your infant's first stools.

Colostrum comes out in small amounts compared to later breast milk, which will fill the alveoli (milk ducts) of your breasts about three days after birth. You'll know when your milk comes in—your breasts will become engorged with milk, be rock hard, and feel sore to the touch. Nursing your baby will relieve the pressure quickly, although it's possible you will need a little additional help to ease soreness. A few clinical studies have shown some benefit in the use of cabbage leaves to relieve the discomfort of engorgement. Massage and warm compresses can also help.

Latching and Letdown

Some babies seem to be breastfeeding champs from the get-go, while others need a little coaching. You're both new at this, so have patience and remember that you'll get better with practice. If you're having a hospital stay after your birth, the nurses on the maternity ward can give you some pointers on technique and check baby's latch. In some cases there will be a lactation specialist on staff to consult with.

Start with a comfortable position for the two of you. Baby's whole body should face yours, not just her turned head. The cradle and cross-cradle holds are two common positions. The cradle holds your baby close across the front of your body, with her head in the crook of your arm and your hand supporting her bottom. The cross-cradle switches arms and puts your hand under her head. Lying down with baby facing you is a good choice for the utterly exhausted.

ESSENTIAL

Sore or dry and cracked nipples are common phenomena as you get on the breastfeeding launch pad. Never fear—they will toughen up. In the meantime, try vitamin E oil for moisturizing or a vegan ointment for easing abrasions and pain. You'll only need a tiny dollop with each.

The football position (or clutch hold) tucks baby under your arm, again facing your body and breast. If you've had a C-section, this can help by keeping the weight off your incision. It's also a favorite of moms with twins who are doing double nursing duty. With all nursing positions, make sure your baby's head is well supported.

After you're settled into position, brace your breast with one hand, cupped in the shape of a *"C."* If you have small breasts, this may not be necessary after a time, but try the C hold initially to make sure baby latches on correctly.

Encouraging baby to get a successful latch is the most important part of the process. Stroke her bottom lip with your nipple until she opens her mouth wide. This is called the *rooting reflex*. Insert your nipple into her mouth, and she should instinctively latch onto it.

A proper latch:

❑ Encompasses the entire nipple and most if not all of the areola.

❑ Positions baby's nose almost directly on your breast. (Don't worry, she can breathe.)

❑ Can be verified by her visible and possibly audible swallowing.

❑ Will *not* hurt (unless the nipple is in poor condition to begin with).

As your baby nurses, you'll feel a warm tingling that signals the milk ejection reflex (MER) or letdown. The sensation is actually that of milk being released into the sinuses of the breast for easy access by baby. Some women don't always feel the MER, but you'll know that it occurs when your baby suddenly picks up his pace of sucking and swallowing.

Supply and Demand System

When the process operates as designed, the more baby nurses, the more milk your breasts produce. A breast that baby has completely drained will produce milk at a faster rate than one that has only been partially emptied. Your milk production takes its cue from baby. So if your child is premature or ill and isn't nursing or is latching or sucking ineffectively, your milk supply will adjust downward. A breast pump can help keep the milk flowing until baby is ready to nurse full time again.

QUESTION

I feel like I'm nursing constantly! Is she not getting enough food? Newborns don't believe much in schedules. In some cases constant nursing in a fussy baby can indicate an insufficient milk supply. But as long as she's growing fine and is having six to eight wet diapers and about three dirty diapers daily, you can be assured she's getting plenty to eat.

Nursing ten to twelve times a day is normal for a newborn. That may seem like a lot, but just bear with it; as the weeks pass and he develops, he'll spend more time exploring and less time eating. In the meantime, his frequent snacks are helping to establish and grow your milk supply, which is great.

Practical Matters

Button-up blouses, shirts with zippers, and other easy-access clothing make nursing easier on a day-to-day basis. There are a variety of nursing bras available; make sure you try them on before purchase to ensure a good fit. You might opt for the comfort of a simple jogging or sports bra that slides up easily, especially if you like the added support of wearing a bra to bed.

Nursing pads for catching leaks before they soak through your shirt are also a must. These come in several different materials and configurations, including cloth, plastic, and disposable. Disposable has the advantage of high absorbency, while cloth can be washed and reused. Accidents do happen, even with pads, and carrying an extra shirt in your bag or car can save you a mortifying moment or two.

Baby's Body and Breastfeeding

Trying to impose a strict feeding schedule on your newborn will result in much heartache and little success. Unless you have multiples, there's really no good reason to start scheduling baby's meals at specific times. If you do have twins or more, you may want to wake them all when one gets up for a feeding in order to get them on a similar routine—but that still doesn't mean feeding by the clock. Only your baby can determine how much she needs to satisfy her tummy, and feeding on demand is the best way to accomplish this.

So how long do you breastfeed? From a clinical standpoint, the American Academy of Pediatrics (AAP) has recommended exclusive breastfeeding for at least six months and promotes breastfeeding for a year or longer, as long as both mother and child are still comfortable with the arrangement. The best answer is probably as long as both of you are still enjoying and benefiting from it.

Bottle Basics

If you do choose to bottle feed, there are literally hundreds of bottle types and nipple configurations on the market to choose from. Figuring out what works and what doesn't is largely trial and error, but there are some factors you can look for. Designs that can be de-aired prior to feeding or that allow an even flow of liquid can reduce baby's gas. Choose a bottle with minimal parts that looks relatively easy to clean and sterilize. If saving time is a priority, features like presterilized disposable bag bottles are a big plus.

Make sure to start baby with a newborn-style nipple that has a smaller opening so she doesn't face a formula tidal wave. If her sucking reflex is weak, however, you might have to upgrade to a larger opening.

Both breastfed and bottle-fed babies require regular burping during a meal. You'll quickly pick up your child's cues that a bubble needs bursting;

she may arch her back and fuss at the breast or bottle. In the beginning, burping at least twice during a feeding session can help ensure her comfort.

ESSENTIAL

Every nursing mother could use a good breastfeeding reference book for guidance. *The Womanly Art of Breastfeeding* from LaLeche League International is considered the breastfeeding bible by many. *The Nursing Mother's Companion* (Harvard Common Press) by lactation consultant Kathleen Huggins, RN, MSN, is also a great resource.

An infant's tiny stomach can only hold 2–4 teaspoons of fluid at birth. Spitting up is his signal that the tank is full. Swallowing air and engaging in too much activity with a full tummy can also cause spit up. However, if baby's spit up becomes excessive and forceful (projectile vomiting) or is accompanied by gagging or difficulty swallowing, call your pediatrician immediately. It could be a sign that your baby has a formula intolerance or a gastrointestinal problem.

Especially for Vegan Moms Who Bottle Feed

If you are not breastfeeding, your baby will need to be fed a commercial infant formula. These formulas are designed to be nutritionally similar to breast milk. Standard formulas are either based on cow's milk or on soy. Soy-based formulas are the best option if you prefer to minimize use of animal products. Discuss formula selection with your baby's pediatrician.

Soymilk, rice milk, and other plant milks are not nutritionally adequate for babies and should not be used to replace breast milk or commercial infant formula before baby's first birthday. Other homemade formulas of any sort should not be used because they don't have the right amounts of protein, fat, and many vitamin and minerals.

Vegan Eating Right: For Mom

A pattern of healthy eating in pregnancy will continue to reward you and baby now that you're breastfeeding. Keep up the same routine with healthy food choices and plenty of noncaffeinated fluids (eight to twelve glasses a day). Nursing burns approximately 500 calories per day. Make nutrient-dense choices, including plenty of fruits, vegetables, whole grains, and plant-based protein foods.

ALERT

If baby becomes fussy after nursing, the cause could be something you ate. Spicy foods can be a trigger, but so can less obvious culprits like vegetables in the cabbage family, grains, and citrus fruits. Skin reactions and congestion can also signal a problem. Keep a food diary to track what foods seem to trigger the reaction, and avoid those that seem to cause problems.

Even though you might be tempted to cut calories drastically in order to get your former figure back, now is not the time to crash diet. Losing weight too quickly can release excessive levels of any toxins like pesticides and PCBs that reside in your maternal fat stores, which will consequently pass into breast milk. Also stay away from extremely low-carbohydrate diets right now, since they can cause ketosis, a potential danger to a nursing baby.

Continuing to take your prenatal supplement is a way to ensure you get the vitamins and minerals you need even on days when you have limited time to prepare food. If your supplement does not contain vitamin B_{12}, you will need to use a separate B_{12} supplement or fortified foods in order to be sure your breast milk meets your baby's needs for this essential vitamin.

One expert panel has recommended that breastfeeding women get at least 300 milligrams a day of DHA. Since you're not eating fish, you'll need to rely on a vegan DHA supplement. See Chapter 6 for more information about DHA. In addition, the American Thyroid Association calls for 150 micrograms daily of supplemental iodine when you're breastfeeding. Check your prenatal—it may supply iodine. If it doesn't, talk to your health care provider about an iodine supplement.

On Your Mind

Breastfeeding doesn't come naturally to everyone. Ingrained feelings of self-consciousness about your body, modesty, and discomfort with the process can inhibit your natural inclination to nurse. When efforts don't go according to plan and the nursing relationship isn't thriving, feelings of inadequacy are common. Seeking assistance, either through coaching or supplemental nutrition, is not a sign of failure but rather of dedication to your child. Breastfeeding in any amount is something to take tremendous pride in.

Breasts: From Form to Function

Where is the right setting to nurse? Wherever your baby is hungry. As long as breastfeeding is done as discretely as circumstances warrant, any place that's appropriate to take a baby is the right spot.

The prospect of nursing in public might be worrying you. When the time comes, don't think about your exposure, think only of filling your child's stomach. A baby who's really singing for her supper will probably not give you the time to be modest about it, anyway.

ESSENTIAL

Breastfeeding problems with your first baby may have made you gun shy. The stress of having a firstborn baby coupled with the exhaustion of new motherhood in the past could have sent your body into a tailspin; there's a good chance this time will be different. You have the added benefit of experience on your side, so don't be afraid to try again.

Specially designed nursing blankets can improve your cover if you're really self-conscious, although a receiving blanket over the shoulder works as well. If you do use a nursing blanket, make sure it's comfortable and not too hot for baby.

Support from Family and Friends

Breastfeeding doesn't always come naturally and immediately, particularly for first-time moms. Having the support of your friends and family is really important in making it through those first few uncertain and some-times rocky weeks. Comments like, "Why don't you just give her a bottle?" will do nothing but erode your confidence and stress you out. Get your part-ner's help in deflecting the negativity and justifying your reasons for breast-feeding, and if the bad attitudes continue, just avoid the offender. You don't need it.

A La Leche League group can also be a steadfast source of support and inspiration and, more important, offer guidance for your breastfeeding dif-ficulties. Call 1-800-LALECHE for a group in your area or see Appendix A for further contact information.

Lactation Problems

Learning to read baby's body language and hear vocal cues is an acquired art, one that takes time to acclimate to. It's easy to miss hunger signals or mistake them for other needs. For now, familiarize yourself with the warn-ing signs of insufficient feeding. If your baby is having fewer than six wet and three dirty diapers a day, is excessively fussy at the breast, has a sunken fontanel (soft spot), acts lethargic, and is not at or above birth weight by two weeks postpartum (or steadily gaining thereafter), he is probably not get-ting enough milk and needs to see his pediatrician immediately. Fortunately, with some work and a little guidance, you should both be able to get back on track.

Why Your Body Isn't Cooperating

There are dozens of reasons why milk supply or nursing itself may not be making the cut, but most of them can be overcome with patience, special equipment, and/or professional training and guidance.

One of the most common reasons for difficulty with nursing is stress. New motherhood and all its related stressors can inhibit milk supply, and tension can make letdown (milk ejection) difficult. If you're uptight about nursing problems, the cycle perpetuates itself. Try to look forward to nursing as a relaxing, destressing time. Poor technique can also cause difficulties. Letting baby empty one breast before moving on to the next will stimulate milk supply and allow her to reach the fatty and filling hindmilk at the end of her drink.

A lactation professional may determine that you have inverted nipples, which make it difficult to achieve a good latch. Breast shields designed to pull the nipple out can help. Breast surgery (enlargement or reduction) can hinder your milk supply. Talk to your doctor if you've had breast surgery and are having lactation problems.

Medications, including some over-the-counter products, can affect your milk supply. Be sure to clear any medication use (prescription or nonprescription) with your doctor if you are breastfeeding.

The mechanics of drinking from a bottle are very different from those of feeding from the breast. If a bottle is introduced before breastfeeding is well established, it's possible for your baby to develop a preference for it.

Babies born prematurely, those with a poor sucking reflex, or those with a cleft lip or other health problem can have problems nursing initially. If your baby needs supplemental feeding in the hospital for any reason, you can request that it be administered with an eyedropper, syringe, feeding cup, or supplemental feeding system to avoid nipple confusion. You should also talk with your pediatrician and a lactation consultant about adaptive techniques and other options.

Lactation Consultants

A lactation consultant is a health care provider who specializes in breastfeeding support and training. If you're having difficulties with nursing, a consultant can be huge in helping you overcome breastfeeding difficulties. Your ob-gyn or your child's pediatrician can provide a referral if needed. Some large pediatric practices retain lactation consultants on staff.

A board-certified lactation consultant will have the designation IBCLC (International Board-Certified Lactation Consultant) or RLC (Registered Lactation Consultant). These mean she meets specific eligibility and experience requirements and has passed a board examination administered by the International Board of Lactation Consultant Examiners (IBLCE). Sometimes consultants are nurses who have earned board certification.

Many certified lactation consultants are also La Leche League leaders. Don't overlook the value of La Leche League support if you have no lactation consultant in your area. The organization can be a tremendous source of emotional support as well as practical advice and expertise.

Pump Primer

A breast pump can be useful in ramping up your milk production if you're having supply issues. It's also a great tool for moms heading back to work who want to keep nursing, as well as for mothers of babies who are temporarily unable to nurse for various health reasons.

A pump may be manual (hand powered), battery powered, or an electrical unit. The hand-powered pumps have the advantage of being inexpensive and portable but can take some getting used to and take longer to empty a breast. They use a piston-like action or a squeeze bulb to create the suction that removes the milk from your breast.

Hospital-grade electric units are probably the most efficient and allow you to pump both breasts at the same time, though they are bulky to transport and costly to purchase. Weekly or monthly rental units are frequently available through lactation consultants, hospital programs, or private businesses. For safety reasons, you will have to purchase a personal kit for use with the rental unit that contains all the elements that come in contact with your breast milk, including tubing and bottles. The kit can be used for as long as you plan to pump.

Supplemental Feeding

If you're having breastfeeding problems, a supplemental nursing system (SNS) can help you provide baby with added nutrients of pumped breast milk or formula while still giving the benefits of suckling. A bottle or bag milk reservoir hangs around your neck, and two narrow silicone tubes channel milk flow from the reservoir to your nipple, where the open end of the tube is taped. As baby feeds on both the supplemental milk and breast milk you're providing, his suckling action further stimulates your milk production.

Women who are having problems producing enough milk for whatever reason may be able to supplement from a local breast milk bank if one is nearby. Milk donors are screened for health problems in a process similar to blood-donation screening. Again, a lactation consultant or pediatrician should have further information on what's available in your area.

Mastitis

Mastitis is an infection of the breast that can be caused by a plugged milk duct. If you develop mastitis, you can and should keep nursing. Your baby cannot get ill, and the breastfeeding process will actually help the mastitis resolve itself faster by easing the pain and draining the milk ducts. Signs of mastitis include:

- Breast is warm to the touch
- Red, tender streaks on the breast
- Pain and swelling
- Fever

If you develop mastitis, stay on your nursing schedule and try to get sufficient rest to help your body heal. A warm water bottle, warm wet compress, or soak in a hot shower can help to ease the discomfort. If the mastitis doesn't start to clear up in a day or so or begins to worsen, you might need an antibiotic. Your health care provider can advise you as to what medications will be safe for breastfeeding.

CHAPTER 17

Vegan Breakfasts

Carob-Peanut Butter-Banana Smoothie

Yummy enough for a dessert but healthy enough for breakfast, this smoothie is also a great protein boost. Grab a whole-grain muffin and you have breakfast to go.

INGREDIENTS | SERVES 2

7–8 ice cubes

2 bananas

2 tablespoons peanut butter

2 tablespoons carob powder

1 cup soymilk

Place all ingredients in a blender and blend together until smooth.

PER SERVING Calories: 262 | Fat: 10g | Sodium: 136mg | Fiber: 6g | Protein: 9g

Strawberry Smoothie

Add silken tofu to a simple fruit smoothie for a creamy protein boost.

INGREDIENTS | SERVES 2

½ cup frozen strawberries (or other berries)

½ block silken tofu

1 banana

¾ cup orange juice

3–4 ice cubes

1 tablespoon agave nectar (optional)

Place all ingredients in a blender and blend together until smooth and creamy.

PER SERVING Calories: 154 | Fat: 3g | Sodium: 6mg | Fiber: 3g | Protein: 5g

Vanilla-Date Breakfast Smoothie

Adding dates to a basic soymilk and fruit smoothie adds a blast of unexpected sweetness. A healthy breakfast treat or a cooling summer snack.

INGREDIENTS | SERVES 1

4 dates
Water, to cover dates
¾ cup soymilk
2 bananas
6–7 ice cubes
¼ teaspoon vanilla

1. Cover the dates with water and allow to soak for at least 10 minutes.

2. Discard the soaking water and add the dates and all other ingredients to the blender.

3. Process on medium until smooth, about 1 minute.

> **PER SERVING** Calories: 439 | Fat: 4g | Sodium: 93mg | Fiber: 11g | Protein: 9g

For a Smoother Smoothie

Soaking your dates first will help them process a little quicker and results in a smoother consistency. Place dates in a small bowl and cover with water. Let them sit for about 10 minutes, then drain.

Peanut Butter Granola Wrap

Eating on the go? This wrap has all you need for a healthy breakfast, including whole grains, fresh fruit, and protein. It's the perfect breakfast for the busy health nut!

INGREDIENTS | SERVES 1

2 tablespoons peanut butter (or other nut butter)
1 whole-wheat flour tortilla
2 tablespoons granola (or any vegan breakfast cereal)
½ banana, sliced thin
¼ teaspoon cinnamon
1 tablespoon raisins
1 teaspoon agave nectar (optional)

1. Spread peanut butter down the center of the tortilla and layer granola and banana on top.

2. Sprinkle with cinnamon and raisins and drizzle with agave nectar if desired.

3. Warm in the microwave for 10–15 seconds to slightly melt peanut butter.

> **PER SERVING** Calories: 423 | Fat: 21g | Sodium: 368mg | Fiber: 8g | Protein: 13g

Quick Tofu Breakfast Burrito

Toss in a fresh diced chili if you need something to really wake you up in the morning.
There's no reason you can't enjoy these burritos for lunch, either!

INGREDIENTS | SERVES 4

1 block (14–16 ounces) firm or extra-firm tofu, well pressed
2 tablespoons olive oil
½ cup salsa
½ teaspoon chili powder
Salt and pepper, to taste
4 flour tortillas, warmed
Ketchup or hot sauce, to taste
4 slices vegan cheese
1 avocado, sliced

1. Cube or crumble the tofu into 1" chunks. Sauté in olive oil over medium heat for 2–3 minutes.

2. Add salsa and chili powder, and cook for 2–3 more minutes, stirring frequently. Season generously with salt and pepper.

3. Layer each warmed tortilla with ¼ of the tofu and salsa mix and drizzle with ketchup or hot sauce.

4. Add vegan cheese and avocado slices and wrap like a burrito.

PER SERVING Calories: 495 | Fat: 29g | Sodium: 626mg | Fiber: 8g | Protein: 24g

Apple Cinnamon Waffles

For perfect vegan waffles, make sure your waffle iron is hot and very well greased,
as vegan waffles tend to be stickier than nonvegan waffles.

INGREDIENTS | SERVES 4

1¼ cups flour
2 teaspoons baking powder
½ teaspoon cinnamon
2 teaspoons sugar
1 cup soymilk
½ cup applesauce
1 teaspoon vanilla
1 tablespoon vegetable oil

1. In a large bowl, combine the flour, baking powder, cinnamon, and sugar. Set aside.

2. In a separate bowl, combine soymilk, applesauce, vanilla, and oil.

3. Add the soymilk mixture to the dry ingredients, stirring just until combined; do not overmix.

4. Carefully drop about ¼ cup batter onto preheated waffle iron for each waffle, and cook until done.

PER SERVING Calories: 230 | Fat: 5g | Sodium: 270mg | Fiber: 2g | Protein: 6g

Granola Breakfast Parfait

Sneak some healthy flax meal or wheat germ into your morning meal by adding it to a layered soy yogurt and granola parfait. If you don't have fresh fruit on hand, try adding some dried fruit, such as chopped dried apricots or pineapple. Serve in glass bowls or cups for presentation.

INGREDIENTS | SERVES 2

¼ cup flax meal or wheat germ

2 containers (6-ounces) soy yogurt, any flavor

2 tablespoons maple syrup or agave nectar (optional)

½ cup granola

½ cup sliced fruit

1. In a small bowl, combine the flax meal or wheat germ, yogurt, and maple syrup.

2. In two serving bowls, place a few spoonfuls of granola, then a layer of soy yogurt. Top with a layer of fresh fruit, and continue layering until ingredients are used up. Serve immediately.

PER SERVING Calories: 354 | Fat: 10g | Sodium: 40mg | Fiber: 8g | Protein: 10g

Maple-Cinnamon Breakfast Quinoa

Quinoa is a filling and healthy breakfast and has more protein than regular oatmeal. This is a deliciously sweet and energizing way to kick off your day.

INGREDIENTS | SERVES 4

1 cup quinoa

2–2½ cups water

1 teaspoon vegan margarine

⅔ cup soymilk

½ teaspoon cinnamon

2 tablespoons maple syrup

2 tablespoons raisins (optional)

2 bananas, sliced (optional)

1. In a small saucepan, bring the quinoa and water to a boil. Reduce to a simmer and allow to cook, covered, for 15 minutes, until liquid is absorbed.

2. Remove from heat and fluff the quinoa with a fork. Cover, and allow to sit for 5 minutes.

3. Stir in the margarine and soymilk, then remaining ingredients.

PER SERVING Calories: 208 | Fat: 4g | Sodium: 39mg | Fiber: 4g | Protein: 7g

No-Sugar Apricot Applesauce

You don't really need to peel the apples if you're short on time, but it only takes about 5 minutes and will give you a smoother sauce. Try adding a touch of nutmeg or pumpkin pie spice for extra flavor.

INGREDIENTS | YIELDS 4 CUPS

6 apples
⅓ cup water
½ cup dried apricots, chopped
4 dates, chopped
Cinnamon, to taste (optional)

1. Peel, core, and chop apples.

2. In a large soup or stock pot, add apples and water and bring to a low boil. Simmer, covered, for 15 minutes, stirring occasionally.

3. Add chopped apricots and dates; simmer for another 10–15 minutes.

4. Mash with a large fork until desired consistency is reached, or allow to cool slightly and purée in a blender until smooth.

5. Sprinkle with cinnamon, to taste.

PER ½ CUP Calories: 109 | Fat: 0g | Sodium: 1mg | Fiber: 2g | Protein: 1g

Fat-Free Banana Bread

You can add ½ cup chopped walnuts to this simple banana bread, but then, of course, it won't be fat free. If you want a bit of texture without the fat, try adding chopped dates or raisins instead.

INGREDIENTS | YIELDS 1 LOAF

4 ripe bananas
⅓ cup soymilk
⅔ cup sugar
1 teaspoon vanilla
2 cups all-purpose flour
1 teaspoon baking powder
½ teaspoon baking soda
½ teaspoon salt
¾ teaspoon cinnamon

1. Preheat oven to 350°F. Lightly grease a loaf pan.

2. Mix together the bananas, soymilk, sugar, and vanilla until smooth and creamy.

3. In a separate bowl, combine the flour, baking powder, baking soda, and salt.

4. Combine the flour mixture with the banana mixture just until smooth.

5. Spread batter in loaf pan and sprinkle the top with cinnamon. Bake for 55 minutes, or until a toothpick inserted in the middle comes out clean.

PER ⅛ LOAF Calories: 237 | Fat: 0g | Sodium: 288mg | Fiber: 3g | Protein: 4g

Quick and Easy Vegan Biscuits

Serve warm from the oven with apple butter or your favorite jam.

INGREDIENTS | YIELDS 12–14 BISCUITS

2 cups flour
1 tablespoon baking powder
½ teaspoon salt
5 tablespoons cold vegan margarine
⅔ cup unsweetened soymilk

1. Preheat oven to 425°F.

2. Combine flour, baking powder, and salt in a large bowl. Add margarine.

3. Using a fork, mash the margarine with the dry ingredients until crumbly.

4. Add soymilk a few tablespoons at a time; combine just until dough forms. You may need to add a little more or less than ⅔ cup.

5. Knead a few times on a floured surface, then roll out to ¾" thick. Cut into 3" rounds.

6. Bake for 12–14 minutes, or until done.

PER 1 BISCUIT Calories: 125 | Fat: 5g | Sodium: 211mg | Fiber: 1g | Protein: 3g

Vanilla Flax Granola

Making your own granola allows you to create whatever flavors you desire.

INGREDIENTS | YIELDS 2½ CUPS

⅔ cup maple syrup
⅓ cup vegan margarine
1½ teaspoons vanilla
2 cups oats
½ cup flax meal or wheat germ
¾ cup dried fruit, small dices

1. Preheat oven to 325°F.

2. Over low heat, melt and whisk together maple syrup, margarine, and vanilla until margarine is melted.

3. Toss together oats, flax meal, and fruit on a large baking tray in a single layer (you may need to use 2 trays).

4. Drizzle maple syrup mixture over oats and fruit; gently toss to combine.

5. Bake for 25–30 minutes, carefully tossing once during cooking. Granola will harden as it cools.

PER ½ CUP Calories: 340 | Fat: 15g | Sodium: 148mg | Fiber: 6g | Protein: 6g

Morning Cereal Bars

Store-bought breakfast bars are often loaded with artificial sugars, and most homemade recipes require corn syrup. This healthier method makes a sweet and filling snack or breakfast to munch on the run.

INGREDIENTS | YIELDS 12–14 BARS

3 cups vegan breakfast cereal, any kind

1 cup peanut butter

⅓ cup tahini

1 cup maple syrup

½ teaspoon vanilla

2 cups muesli

½ cup flax meal or wheat germ

½ cup diced dried fruit or raisins

1. Lightly grease a baking pan or 2 casserole pans.

2. Place cereal in a sealable bag and crush partially with a rolling pin. If you're using a smaller cereal, you can skip this step. Set aside.

3. Combine peanut butter, tahini, and maple syrup in a large saucepan over low heat, stirring well to combine.

4. Remove from heat and stir in the vanilla, then the cereal, muesli, flax meal or wheat germ, and dried fruit or raisins.

5. Press firmly into greased baking pan and chill until firm, about 45 minutes. Slice into bars.

PER 1 BAR Calories: 326 | Fat: 15g | Sodium: 194mg | Fiber: 3g | Protein: 8g

Sweet Potato Apple Latkes

Serve topped with No-Sugar Apricot Applesauce (Chapter 17) or nondairy sour cream.

INGREDIENTS | YIELDS 1 DOZEN LATKES

3 large sweet potatoes, grated

1 apple, grated

1 small yellow onion, grated

Egg replacer for 2 eggs

3 tablespoons flour

1 teaspoon baking powder

½ teaspoon cinnamon

½ teaspoon nutmeg

½ teaspoon salt

Oil for frying

1. Using a cloth or paper towel, gently squeeze out excess moisture from potatoes and apples; combine with onions in a large bowl.

2. Mix together remaining ingredients except oil; combine with potato mixture.

3. In a skillet or frying pan, heat a few tablespoons of oil. Drop potato mixture in the hot oil a scant ¼ cup at a time. Use a spatula to flatten, forming a pancake. Cook for 3–4 minutes on each side, until lightly crisped.

PER 1 LATKE Calories: 89 | Fat: 4g | Sodium: 162mg | Fiber: 2g | Protein: 1g

Super Green Quiche

Get your greens in before noon with this veggie quiche.

INGREDIENTS | SERVES 4

1 (10-ounce) package frozen chopped spinach, thawed and drained

½ cup broccoli, diced small

1 block (14–16 ounces) firm or extra-firm tofu

1 tablespoon soy sauce

¼ cup soymilk

1 teaspoon prepared mustard

2 tablespoons nutritional yeast

½ teaspoon garlic powder

1 teaspoon parsley

½ teaspoon rosemary

¾ teaspoon salt

¼ teaspoon pepper

Prepared vegan crust

1. Preheat oven to 350°F.

2. Steam the spinach and broccoli until just lightly cooked, then set aside to cool. Press as much moisture as possible out of the spinach.

3. In a blender or food processor, combine the tofu with the remaining ingredients except crust until well mixed. Mix in the spinach and broccoli by hand until combined.

4. Spread mixture evenly in pie crust.

5. Bake for 35–40 minutes, or until firm. Allow to cool for at least 10 minutes before serving. Quiche will firm up a bit more as it cools.

PER SERVING Calories: 403 | Fat: 20g | Sodium: 1,560mg | Fiber: 7g | Protein: 17g

Vegan Pancakes

A touch of sugar and hint of sweet banana flavor make this pancake recipe sparkle.

INGREDIENTS | YIELDS 1 DOZEN PANCAKES

1 cup flour

1 tablespoon sugar

1¾ teaspoons baking powder

¼ teaspoon salt

½ banana

1 teaspoon vanilla

1 cup soymilk

1. In a large bowl, mix together flour, sugar, baking powder, and salt.

2. In a separate small bowl, mash banana with a fork. Add vanilla; whisk until smooth and fluffy. Add soymilk; stir to combine well.

3. Add wet mixture to dry ingredients; stir.

4. Heat a lightly greased griddle or large frying pan over medium heat. Drop batter about 3 tablespoons at a time and heat until bubbles appear on surface, about 2–3 minutes. Flip and cook other side until lightly golden brown, another 1–2 minutes.

PER 1 PANCAKE Calories: 56 | Fat: 0g | Sodium: 128mg | Fiber: 0g | Protein: 2g

Baked "Sausage" and Mushroom Frittata

Baked tofu frittatas are an easy brunch or weekend breakfast. Once you've got the technique down, it's easy to adjust the ingredients to your liking. With tofu and mock meat, this one packs a super protein punch!

INGREDIENTS | SERVES 4

½ yellow onion, diced

3 cloves garlic, minced

½ cup sliced mushrooms

1 (12-ounce) package vegetarian sausage substitute or vegetarian "beef" crumbles

2 tablespoons olive oil

¾ teaspoon salt, or to taste

¼ teaspoon black pepper

1 block (14–16 ounces) firm or extra-firm tofu

1 block (approximately 12 ounces) silken tofu

1 tablespoon soy sauce

2 tablespoons nutritional yeast

¼ teaspoon turmeric (optional)

1 tomato, sliced thin (optional)

1. Preheat oven to 325°F and lightly grease a glass pie pan.

2. In a large skillet, heat onion, garlic, mushrooms, and vegetarian sausage in olive oil until sausage is browned and mushrooms are soft, about 3–4 minutes. Season with salt and pepper and set aside.

3. Combine firm tofu, silken tofu, soy sauce, nutritional yeast, and turmeric in a blender; process until mixed. Combine tofu mixture with sausage mixture; spread into pan. Layer slices of tomato on top (optional).

4. Bake in oven for about 45 minutes, or until firm. Allow to cool for 5–10 minutes before serving, as frittata will set as it cools.

PER SERVING Calories: 301 | Fat: 17g | Sodium: 1,037mg | Fiber: 4g | Protein: 25g

Chili Masala Tofu Scramble

Tofu scramble is an easy and versatile vegan breakfast. This version adds chili and curry for continental flavor. Toss in whatever veggies you have on hand—tomatoes, spinach, or diced broccoli would work well.

INGREDIENTS | SERVES 4

1 block (14–16 ounces) firm or extra-firm tofu, pressed
1 small onion, diced
2 cloves garlic, minced
2 tablespoons olive oil
1 small red chili pepper, minced
1 green bell pepper, chopped
¾ cup sliced mushrooms
1 tablespoon soy sauce
1 teaspoon curry powder
½ teaspoon cumin
¼ teaspoon turmeric
1 teaspoon nutritional yeast (optional)

1. Cut pressed tofu into 1" cubes or crumble into medium-small pieces.

2. Sauté onion and garlic in olive oil until onions are soft, about 1–2 minutes.

3. Add tofu, chili pepper, bell pepper, and mushrooms, stirring well to combine.

4. Add remaining ingredients, except nutritional yeast, and combine well. Allow to cook until tofu is lightly browned, about 6–8 minutes.

5. Remove from heat and stir in nutritional yeast if desired.

PER SERVING Calories: 144 | Fat: 10g | Sodium: 240mg | Fiber: 2g | Protein: 8g

The Next Day

Leftover tofu scramble makes an excellent lunch, or wrap leftovers in a warmed flour tortilla to make breakfast-style burritos, perhaps with some salsa or beans. Why isn't it called scrambled tofu instead of tofu scramble if it's a substitute for scrambled eggs? This is one of the great conundrums of veganism.

Easy Vegan French Toast

For a leisurely weekend breakfast, try golden-fried French toast topped with a fruit compote or some agave nectar or maple syrup.

INGREDIENTS | SERVES 4

2 bananas

½ cup soymilk

1 tablespoon orange juice

1 tablespoon maple syrup

¾ teaspoon vanilla

1 tablespoon flour

1 teaspoon cinnamon

½ teaspoon nutmeg

Oil or vegan margarine, for frying

12 thick slices bread

The Perfect Vegan French Toast

Creating an eggless French toast is a true art. Is your French toast too soggy or too dry? Thickly sliced bread lightly toasted will be more absorbent. Too mushy, or the mixture doesn't want to stick? Try spooning it onto your bread, rather than dipping.

1. Using a blender or mixer, mix together the bananas, soymilk, orange juice, maple syrup, and vanilla until smooth and creamy.

2. Whisk in flour, cinnamon, and nutmeg; pour into a pie plate or shallow pan.

3. In a large skillet, heat 1–2 tablespoons of vegan margarine or oil.

4. Dip or spoon mixture over each bread slice on both sides and fry in hot oil until lightly golden brown on both sides, about 2–3 minutes.

PER SERVING Calories: 391 | Fat: 11g | Sodium: 629mg | Fiber: 4g | Protein: 9g

Whole-Wheat Blueberry Muffins

Because these muffins have very little fat, they'll want to stick to the papers or the muffin tin. Letting them cool before removing them will help prevent this, and be sure to grease your muffin tin well.

INGREDIENTS | YIELDS APPROX. 1½ DOZEN MUFFINS

2 cups whole-wheat flour

1 cup all-purpose flour

1¼ cups sugar

1 tablespoon baking powder

1 teaspoon salt

1½ cups soymilk

½ cup applesauce

½ teaspoon vanilla

2 cups blueberries

Making Vegan Muffins

Got a favorite muffin recipe? Try making it vegan! Use a commercial egg replacer in place of the eggs, and substitute a vegan soy margarine and soymilk for the butter and milk. Voilà!

1. Preheat oven to 400°F.

2. In a large bowl, combine the flours, sugar, baking powder, and salt. Set aside.

3. In a separate small bowl, whisk together the soymilk, applesauce, and vanilla until well mixed.

4. Combine the wet ingredients with the dry ingredients; stir just until mixed. Gently fold in ½ of the blueberries.

5. Spoon batter into lined or greased muffin tins, filling each tin about ⅔ full. Sprinkle remaining blueberries on top of muffins.

6. Bake for 20–25 minutes, or until lightly golden brown on top.

PER 1 MUFFIN Calories: 147 | Fat: 1g | Sodium: 220mg | Fiber: 2g | Protein: 3g

CHAPTER 18

Entrées

Three-Bean Casserole

If you like baked beans, you'll like this easy bean casserole. It's an easy entrée you can get in the oven in just a few minutes.

INGREDIENTS | SERVES 8

1 (15-ounce) can vegetarian baked beans

1 (15-ounce) can black beans, drained and rinsed

1 (15-ounce) can kidney beans, drained and rinsed

1 onion, chopped

⅓ cup ketchup

3 tablespoons apple cider vinegar

⅓ cup brown sugar

2 teaspoons mustard powder

2 teaspoons garlic powder

4 vegan hot dogs, cooked and chopped (optional)

1. Preheat oven to 350°F.

2. Combine all ingredients except hot dogs in a large casserole dish.

3. Bake, uncovered, for 55 minutes. Add precooked vegan hot dogs just before serving.

PER SERVING Calories: 202 | Fat: 1g | Sodium: 553mg | Fiber: 10g | Protein: 10g

Barley Baked Beans

If you've got a slow cooker, you can dump all the ingredients in and cook it on a medium setting for about 6 hours.

INGREDIENTS | SERVES 8

2 cups cooked barley

2 (15-ounce) cans pinto or navy beans, drained and rinsed

1 onion, diced

1 (28-ounce) can crushed or diced tomatoes

½ cup water

¼ cup brown sugar

⅓ cup barbecue sauce

2 tablespoons molasses

2 teaspoons mustard powder

1 teaspoon garlic powder

1 teaspoon salt, or to taste

1. Preheat oven to 300°F.

2. In a large oiled casserole or baking dish, combine all ingredients. Cover, and bake for 2 hours, stirring occasionally.

3. Uncover and bake for 15 more minutes, or until thick and saucy.

PER SERVING Calories: 224 | Fat: 1g | Sodium: 849mg | Fiber: 9g | Protein: 8g

Chickpea Soft Tacos

For an easy and healthy taco filling wrapped up in flour tortillas, try using chickpeas! Short on time? Pick up taco seasoning packets to use instead of the spice blend—but watch out for added MSG.

INGREDIENTS | SERVES 6

2 (15-ounce) cans chickpeas, drained and rinsed

½ cup water

1 (6-ounce) can tomato paste

1 tablespoon chili powder

1 teaspoon garlic powder

½ teaspoon onion powder

½ teaspoon cumin

¼ cup chopped fresh cilantro (optional)

4 flour tortillas

Optional taco fillings: shredded lettuce, black olives, vegan cheese, nondairy sour cream

1. In a large skillet, combine chickpeas, water, tomato paste, chili, garlic, onion powder, and cumin. Cover and simmer for 10 minutes, stirring occasionally. Uncover and simmer 1–2 minutes, until most of the liquid is absorbed.

2. Use a fork or potato masher to mash the chickpeas until half mashed. Stir in fresh cilantro if desired.

3. Spoon mixture into flour tortillas, add toppings, and wrap.

PER SERVING Calories: 285 | Fat: 4g | Sodium: 641mg | Fiber: 8g | Protein: 11g

Couscous and Bean Pilaf

*A quick lunch or dinner entrée that can be served hot or cold.
Add a few extra veggies for a meal in a bowl.*

INGREDIENTS | SERVES 4

2 cups water or vegetable broth

2 cups couscous

2 tablespoons olive oil

2 tablespoons red wine vinegar

½ teaspoon crushed red pepper flakes

1 (15-ounce) can great northern or cannellini beans, drained and rinsed

2 tablespoons minced pimiento peppers

2 tablespoons chopped fresh parsley

Salt and pepper, to taste

1. Bring the water or vegetable broth to a simmer; add couscous. Cover, turn off heat, and allow to sit for at least 15 minutes to cook couscous. Fluff with a fork.

2. Whisk together the olive oil, vinegar, and pepper flakes; toss with couscous.

3. Combine beans, peppers, and parsley with couscous; toss gently to combine. Season with salt and pepper.

PER SERVING Calories: 509 | Fat: 8g | Sodium: 32mg | Fiber: 10g | Protein: 19g

Italian White Beans and Rice

This is a quick, inexpensive, and hearty meal that will quickly become a favorite standby on busy nights. It's nutritious, filling, and can easily be doubled for a crowd.

INGREDIENTS | SERVES 4

½ onion, diced

2 ribs celery, diced

3 cloves garlic, minced

2 tablespoons olive oil

1 (14-ounce) can diced or crushed tomatoes

1 (15-ounce) can cannellini or great northern beans, drained and rinsed

½ teaspoon parsley

½ teaspoon basil

1 cup rice, cooked

1 tablespoon balsamic vinegar

1. Sauté onion, celery, and garlic in olive oil for 3–5 minutes, until onion and celery are soft.

2. Reduce heat to medium-low and add tomatoes, beans, parsley, and basil. Cover, and simmer for 10 minutes, stirring occasionally.

3. Stir in cooked rice and balsamic vinegar; cook, uncovered, a few more minutes, until liquid is absorbed.

PER SERVING Calories: 325 | Fat: 8g | Sodium: 135mg | Fiber: 8g | Protein: 12g

Macro-Inspired Veggie Bowl

Truly nourishing, this is a full meal in a bowl, inspired by macrobiotic cuisine.

INGREDIENTS | SERVES 6

2 cups brown rice, cooked

1 batch Sesame Baked Tofu (Chapter 18), chopped into cubes

1 head broccoli, steamed and chopped

1 red or yellow bell pepper, sliced thin

1 cup You Are a Goddess Dressing (Chapter 20)

½ cup pumpkin seeds or sunflower seeds

2 teaspoons dulse or kelp seaweed flakes (optional)

1. Divide brown rice into 6 bowls.

2. Top each bowl with Sesame Baked Tofu, broccoli, and bell pepper.

3. Drizzle with dressing, and sprinkle with seeds and seaweed flakes.

PER SERVING Calories: 547 | Fat: 37g | Sodium: 911 | Fiber: 11g | Protein: 28g

Quinoa and Hummus Sandwich Wrap

*Lunch is the perfect time to fill up on whole grains.
If you've got leftover tabbouleh, use that in place of the cooked quinoa.*

INGREDIENTS | SERVES 1

1 tortilla or flavored wrap, warmed

3 tablespoons hummus

⅓ cup cooked quinoa

½ teaspoon lemon juice

2 teaspoons Italian or vinaigrette salad dressing

1 roasted red pepper, sliced into strips

1. Spread warmed tortilla with a layer of hummus, then quinoa; drizzle with lemon juice and salad dressing.

2. Layer red pepper on top; wrap.

PER SERVING Calories: 332 | Fat: 12g | Sodium: 627mg | Fiber: 6g | Protein: 11g

Five-Minute Vegan Pasta Salad

Once you've got the pasta cooked and cooled, this takes just 5 minutes to assemble, as it's made with store-bought dressing. A balsamic vinaigrette or tomato dressing would also work well.

INGREDIENTS | SERVES 4

4 cups pasta, cooked

¾ cup vegan Italian salad dressing

3 scallions, chopped

½ cup sliced black olives

1 tomato, chopped

1 avocado, diced (optional)

Salt and pepper, to taste

Toss together all ingredients. Allow to chill for at least 1½ hours before serving, if time allows, to allow flavors to combine.

PER SERVING Calories: 378 | Fat: 16g | Sodium: 877mg | Fiber: 4g | Protein: 9g

Pasta and Peas

*Great for the kids, but use artichoke hearts or broccoli to make it for adults,
or any frozen mixed veggies you like.*

INGREDIENTS | SERVES 6

1½ cups plain or unsweetened soymilk

1 teaspoon garlic powder

2 tablespoons vegan margarine

1 tablespoon flour

1½ cups green peas, fresh or frozen, thawed

⅓ cup nutritional yeast

1 (12-ounce) package pasta, cooked

Salt and pepper, to taste

1. In a medium pot, whisk together the soymilk, garlic powder, and margarine over low heat. Add flour; stir well to combine, heating just until thickened, about 5 minutes.

2. Add peas and nutritional yeast until heated and well mixed, about 5 minutes; pour over pasta.

3. Season with salt and pepper, to taste.

PER SERVING Calories: 312 | Fat: 6g | Sodium: 124mg | Fiber: 4g | Protein: 13g

Easy Fried Tofu

*A simple fried tofu that you can serve with just about any dipping sauce for a snack,
or add to salads or stir-fries instead of plain tofu.*

INGREDIENTS | SERVES 3

1 block (14–16 ounces) firm or extra-firm tofu, cubed

¼ cup soy sauce (optional)

2 tablespoons flour

2 tablespoons nutritional yeast

1 teaspoon garlic powder

¼ teaspoon salt, or to taste

Dash pepper

Oil for frying

1. Marinate sliced tofu in soy sauce in the refrigerator for at least 1 hour. This step is optional.

2. In a small bowl, combine flour, yeast, garlic powder, salt, and pepper.

3. Coat tofu well with flour mixture on all sides.

4. Fry in hot oil until crispy and lightly golden brown on all sides, about 4–5 minutes.

PER SERVING Calories: 232 | Fat: 19g | Sodium: 208mg | Fiber: 2g | Protein: 11g

Eggless Egg Salad

Vegan egg salad looks just like the real thing and is much quicker to make. Use this recipe to make egg salad sandwiches, or serve it on a bed of lettuce with tomato slices and enjoy it just as it is.

INGREDIENTS | SERVES 4

1 block (14–16 ounces) firm tofu, lightly steamed and cooled

1 (12-ounce) block silken tofu

½ cup vegan mayonnaise

⅓ cup sweet pickle relish

¾ teaspoon apple cider vinegar

½ stalk celery, diced

2 tablespoons minced onion

1½ tablespoons Dijon mustard

2 tablespoons chopped chives (optional)

2 tablespoons vegetarian bacon bits (optional)

1 teaspoon paprika

1. In a medium-size bowl, use a fork to mash the tofu together with the rest of the ingredients, except the bacon bits and paprika.

2. Chill for at least 15 minutes before serving to allow flavors to mingle.

3. Garnish with bacon bits and paprika just before serving.

PER SERVING Calories: 318 | Fat: 24g | Sodium: 428mg | Fiber: 2g | Protein: 11g

Black and Green-Veggie Burritos

Black bean burritos filled with zucchini or yellow summer squash. Just add in the fixings—salsa, avocado slices, some nondairy sour cream—the works!

INGREDIENTS | SERVES 4

1 onion, chopped

2 zucchini or yellow squash, cut into thin strips

1 bell pepper, any color, chopped

2 tablespoons olive oil

½ teaspoon oregano

½ teaspoon cumin

1 (15-ounce) can black beans, drained and rinsed

1 (4-ounce) can green chilies

1 cup cooked rice

4 large flour tortillas, warmed

1. Heat onion, zucchini, and bell pepper in olive oil until vegetables are soft, about 4–5 minutes.

2. Reduce heat to low and add oregano, cumin, black beans, and chilies; combine well. Cook, stirring, until well combined and heated through.

3. Place ¼ cup rice in the center of each flour tortilla and top with the bean mixture. Fold the bottom of the tortilla up, then snugly wrap one side, then the other.

4. Serve as is, or bake in a 350°F oven for 15 minutes for a crispy burrito.

PER SERVING Calories: 377 | Fat: 10g | Sodium: 554mg | Fiber: 13g | Protein: 15g

Barley Pilaf with Edamame and Roasted Red Peppers

Don't forget: Freshly ground pepper will give the best flavor to all your recipes, including this one. Serve chilled like a salad, or heat the edamame lightly first for a warmed and high-protein pilaf.

INGREDIENTS | SERVES 6

2 cups frozen shelled edamame, thawed and drained

2 cups cooked barley

½ cup chopped roasted red peppers

⅔ cup green peas, fresh or frozen, thawed

⅔ cup corn, fresh, canned, or frozen, thawed

1½ tablespoons Dijon mustard

2 tablespoons lemon or lime juice

¾ teaspoon garlic powder

2 tablespoons olive oil

Salt and pepper, to taste

¼ cup chopped fresh cilantro

1 avocado, diced (optional)

1. In a large bowl, combine the edamame, barley, peppers, peas, and corn.

2. In a separate small bowl, whisk together the mustard, lemon or lime juice, garlic powder, and olive oil. Drizzle over barley mixture; toss gently to coat well.

3. Season with salt and pepper and toss lightly with cilantro and avocado.

PER SERVING Calories: 190 | Fat: 4g | Sodium: 100mg | Fiber: 9g | Protein: 9g

Curried Rice and Lentils

With no added fat, this is a very simple one-pot side dish-starter recipe. Personalize it with some chopped greens, browned seitan, or a veggie mix.

INGREDIENTS | SERVES 4

1½ cups white rice, uncooked

1 cup lentils, uncooked

2 tomatoes, diced

3½ cups water or vegetable broth

1 bay leaf (optional)

1 tablespoon curry powder

½ teaspoon cumin

½ teaspoon turmeric

½ teaspoon garlic powder

Salt and pepper, to taste

1. In a large soup or stock pot, combine all ingredients except salt and pepper. Bring to a slow simmer, then cover and cook for 20 minutes, stirring occasionally, until rice is done and liquid is absorbed.

2. Taste, then add salt and pepper as desired. Remove bay leaf before serving.

PER SERVING Calories: 436 | Fat: 1g | Sodium: 13mg | Fiber: 17g | Protein: 18g

Peanut Butter Noodles Not Just for Kids

Drown your noodles in this mildly flavored peanut butter sauce recipe.
Who doesn't love peanut butter?

INGREDIENTS | SERVES 4

1 pound Asian-style noodles or regular pasta

⅓ cup peanut butter

⅓ cup water

3 tablespoons soy sauce

2 tablespoons lime juice

2 tablespoons rice vinegar

1 tablespoon sesame oil

½ teaspoon ginger powder

1 teaspoon sugar

½ teaspoon crushed red pepper flakes (optional)

1. Prepare noodles or pasta according to package instructions and set aside.

2. Whisk together remaining ingredients over low heat just until combined, about 3 minutes. Toss with noodles.

PER SERVING Calories: 584 | Fat: 16g | Sodium: 782mg | Fiber: 5g | Protein: 21g

Balsamic Dijon Orzo

Defying logic, this simple dish flavored with balsamic and Dijon is somehow exponentially greater than the sum of its parts. Add a dash of sugar or agave if you find the tangy Dijon overpowering.

INGREDIENTS | SERVES 4

3 tablespoons balsamic vinegar

1½ tablespoons Dijon mustard

1½ tablespoons olive oil

1 teaspoon basil

1 teaspoon parsley

½ teaspoon oregano

1½ cups orzo, cooked

2 medium tomatoes, chopped

½ cup sliced black olives

1 (15-ounce) can great northern or cannellini beans, drained and rinsed

½ teaspoon salt, or to taste

¼ teaspoon pepper

1. In a small bowl or container, whisk together the vinegar, mustard, olive oil, basil, parsley, and oregano until well mixed.

2. Over low heat, combine the orzo with the balsamic dressing; add tomatoes, olives, and beans. Cook for 3–4 minutes, stirring to combine.

3. Season with salt and pepper.

PER SERVING Calories: 356 | Fat: 8g | Sodium: 505mg | Fiber: 8g | Protein: 14g

Creamy Sun-Dried Tomato Pasta

Silken tofu makes a creamy low-fat sauce base. If using dried tomatoes rather than oil-packed, be sure to rehydrate them well first.

INGREDIENTS | SERVES 6

1 (12-ounce) block silken tofu, drained
¼ cup soymilk
2 tablespoons red wine vinegar
½ teaspoon garlic powder
½ teaspoon salt, or to taste
1¼ cups sun-dried tomatoes, rehydrated
1 teaspoon parsley
1 (12-ounce) package pasta, cooked
2 tablespoons chopped fresh basil

1. In a blender or food processor, blend together the tofu, soymilk, vinegar, garlic powder, and salt until smooth and creamy. Add tomatoes and parsley; pulse until tomatoes are finely diced.

2. Transfer sauce to a small pot and heat over medium-low heat just until hot, about 5–10 minutes.

3. Pour sauce over pasta and sprinkle with fresh chopped basil.

PER SERVING Calories: 274 | Fat: 3g | Sodium: 441mg | Fiber: 3g | Protein: 12g

Lemon Basil Tofu

Moist and chewy, this zesty baked tofu is reminiscent of lemon chicken. Serve over steamed rice with extra marinade.

INGREDIENTS | SERVES 6

3 tablespoons lemon juice
1 tablespoon soy sauce
2 teaspoons apple cider vinegar
1 tablespoon Dijon mustard
¾ teaspoon sugar
3 tablespoons olive oil
2 tablespoons chopped basil, plus extra for garnish
2 blocks (14–16 ounces each) firm or extra-firm tofu, well pressed

1. Whisk together all ingredients except tofu; transfer to a baking dish or casserole pan.

2. Slice the tofu into ½" thick strips or triangles.

3. Place the tofu in the marinade and coat well. Allow to marinate in the refrigerator for at least 1 hour or overnight, being sure tofu is well coated in marinade.

4. Preheat oven to 350°F.

5. Bake for 15 minutes, turn over, then bake for another 10–12 minutes, or until done. Garnish with a few extra bits of chopped fresh basil.

PER SERVING Calories: 143 | Fat: 11g | Sodium: 192mg | Fiber: 1g | Protein: 9g

Mexico City Protein Bowl

*A quick meal in a bowl, reminiscent of Mexico City street food stalls,
but healthier and with less pollution.*

INGREDIENTS | SERVES 2

½ block (7–8 ounces) firm tofu, diced small

1 scallion, chopped

1 tablespoon olive oil

½ cup peas, fresh or frozen, thawed

½ cup corn kernels, fresh, canned, or frozen, thawed

½ teaspoon chili powder

1 (15-ounce) can black beans, drained and rinsed

2 corn tortillas

Hot sauce, to taste

1. Heat tofu and scallion in olive oil for 2–3 minutes; add peas, corn, and chili powder. Cook another 1–2 minutes, stirring frequently.

2. Reduce heat to medium-low; add black beans. Heat for 4–5 minutes, until well combined and heated through.

3. Place a corn tortilla in the bottom of a bowl; spoon ½ the beans and tofu over the top of each. Season with hot sauce, to taste.

PER SERVING Calories: 735 | Fat: 28g | Sodium: 452mg | Fiber: 24g | Protein: 55g

Pineapple-Glazed Tofu

*If you like sweet and sour dishes, try this saucy, sweet, Pineapple-Glazed Tofu, excellent for kids.
Toss with some noodles, or add some diced veggies to make it an entrée.*

INGREDIENTS | SERVES 3

½ cup pineapple preserves

2 tablespoons balsamic vinegar

2 tablespoons soy sauce

⅔ cup pineapple juice

1 block (14–16 ounces) firm or extra-firm tofu, cubed

3 tablespoons flour

2 tablespoons oil

1 teaspoon cornstarch

1. Whisk together the preserves, vinegar, soy sauce, and pineapple juice.

2. Coat tofu in flour, then sauté in oil for 1–2 minutes, until lightly golden.

3. Reduce heat to medium-low; add pineapple sauce, stirring well to combine and coat tofu.

4. Heat for 3–4 minutes, stirring frequently, then add cornstarch, whisking to combine and avoid lumps. Heat for a few more minutes, stirring, until sauce has thickened.

PER SERVING Calories: 360 | Fat: 14g | Sodium: 639mg | Fiber: 2g | Protein: 11g

Tandoori Seitan

You can enjoy the flavors of traditional Indian tandoori without firing up your grill by simmering the seitan on the stove top.

INGREDIENTS | SERVES 6

⅔ cup plain soy yogurt

2 tablespoons lemon juice

1½ tablespoons tandoori spice blend

½ teaspoon cumin

½ teaspoon garlic powder

¼ teaspoon salt, or to taste

1 (16-ounce) package prepared seitan, chopped

1 bell pepper, chopped

1 onion, chopped

1 tomato, chopped

2 tablespoons oil

1. In a shallow bowl or pan, whisk together the yogurt, lemon juice, and all the spices; add seitan. Allow to marinate in the refrigerator for at least 1 hour. Reserve marinade.

2. Sauté pepper, onion, and tomato in oil until just barely soft.

3. Reduce heat to low; add seitan. Cook, tossing seitan occasionally, for 8–10 minutes.

4. Serve topped with extra marinade.

PER SERVING Calories: 148 | Fat: 6g | Sodium: 419mg | Fiber: 2g | Protein: 16g

Stove Top Cheater's Mac 'n' Cheese

Yes, it's cheating just a little to make vegan macaroni and cheese starting with store-bought "cheese," but who cares? The secret to getting this recipe super creamy and cheesy is using cream cheese as well as vegan Cheddar. It's not particularly healthy, but at least it's still cholesterol free!

INGREDIENTS | SERVES 6

1 (12-ounce) package macaroni

1 cup plain or unsweetened soymilk

2 tablespoons vegan margarine

½ teaspoon onion powder

1 teaspoon garlic powder

½ cup vegan cream cheese

½ cup vegan Cheddar cheese, grated

⅓ cup nutritional yeast

½ teaspoon salt, or to taste

Black pepper, to taste

1. Prepare macaroni according to package instructions. Drain well and return to pot.

2. Over low heat, stir in soymilk and vegan margarine until melted.

3. Add remaining ingredients, stirring to combine over low heat, until cheese is melted and ingredients are well mixed, about 5–10 minutes.

PER SERVING Calories: 411 | Fat: 13g | Sodium: 549mg | Fiber: 3g | Protein: 13g

Sweet and Spicy Peanut Noodles

*Like the call of the siren, these noodles entice you with their sweet pineapple flavor,
then scorch your tongue with fiery chilies. Very sneaky, indeed.*

INGREDIENTS | SERVES 4

1 (12-ounce) package Asian-style noodles

⅓ cup peanut butter

2 tablespoons soy sauce

⅔ cup pineapple juice

2 cloves garlic, minced

1 teaspoon fresh ginger, grated

½ teaspoon salt, or to taste

1 tablespoon olive oil

1 teaspoon sesame oil

2–3 small chilies, minced

¾ cup diced pineapple, fresh or canned

1. Prepare noodles according to package instructions and set aside.

2. In a small saucepan over low heat, stir together the peanut butter, soy sauce, pineapple juice, garlic, ginger, and salt just until well combined, about 5 minutes.

3. In a large skillet, heat the oils; fry chilies and pineapple, stirring frequently, until pineapple is lightly browned, about 2–3 minutes,. Add noodles; fry for another minute, stirring well.

4. Reduce heat to low and add peanut butter sauce mixture; stir to combine well. Heat for 1 more minute.

PER SERVING Calories: 329 | Fat: 16g | Sodium: 977mg | Fiber: 2g | Protein: 10g

Pineapple TVP Baked Beans

*Add a kick to these saucy homemade vegetarian baked beans
with a bit of cayenne pepper if you'd like.*

INGREDIENTS | SERVES 4

2 (15-ounce) cans pinto or navy beans, partially drained

1 onion, diced

⅔ cup vegan barbecue sauce

2 tablespoons prepared mustard

2 tablespoons brown sugar

1 cup TVP

1 cup hot water

1 (8-ounce) can diced pineapple, drained

¾ teaspoon salt, or to taste

½ teaspoon pepper

1. In a large stock pot, combine beans and about half their liquid, onion, barbecue sauce, mustard, and brown sugar; bring to a slow simmer. Cover and allow to cook for at least 10 minutes, stirring occasionally.

2. Combine TVP with hot water; allow to sit for 6–8 minutes to rehydrate TVP. Drain.

3. Add TVP, pineapple, salt, and pepper to beans; cover and slowly simmer another 10–12 minutes.

PER SERVING Calories: 389 | Fat: 2g | Sodium: 1,461mg | Fiber: 15g | Protein: 23g

Tofu "Chicken" Nuggets

Try dipping these nuggets into ketchup or a sweet and sour sauce.

INGREDIENTS | SERVES 4

¼ cup plain or unsweetened soymilk

2 tablespoons prepared mustard

3 tablespoons nutritional yeast

½ cup bread crumbs

½ cup flour

1 teaspoon poultry seasoning

1 teaspoon garlic powder

1 teaspoon onion powder

½ teaspoon salt, or to taste

¼ teaspoon pepper

1 block (14–16 ounces) firm or extra-firm tofu, sliced into thin strips

Oil for frying (optional)

1. In a large shallow pan, whisk together the soymilk, mustard, and nutritional yeast.

2. In a separate bowl, combine the bread crumbs, flour, poultry seasoning, garlic, onion powder, salt, and pepper.

3. Coat each piece of tofu with the soymilk mixture, then coat well in bread crumbs and flour mixture.

4. Fry in hot oil until lightly golden browned, about 3–4 minutes on each side, or bake in 375°F oven for 20 minutes, turning once.

PER SERVING Calories: 131 | Fat: 5g | Sodium: 492mg | Fiber: 2g | Protein: 10g

The Easiest Black Bean Burger Recipe in the World

Veggie burgers are notorious for falling apart. If you're sick of crumbly burgers, try this simple method for making black bean patties. It's 100 percent guaranteed to stick together.

INGREDIENTS | YIELDS 6 PATTIES

1 (15-ounce) can black beans, drained and rinsed

3 tablespoons minced onions

1 teaspoon salt, or to taste

1½ teaspoons garlic powder

2 teaspoons parsley

1 teaspoon chili powder

⅔ cup flour

Oil for pan frying

1. In a blender or food processor, process the black beans until halfway mashed, or mash with a fork.

2. Remove to a bowl and add onions, salt, garlic powder, parsley, and chili powder and mash to combine.

3. Add flour, a bit at time, again mashing together to combine. You may need a little bit more or less than ⅔ cup. Beans should stick together completely.

4. Form into patties and pan fry in a bit of oil for 2–3 minutes on each side. Patties will appear to be done on the outside while still a bit mushy on the inside, so fry them a few minutes longer than you think they need.

PER 1 PATTY Calories: 210 | Fat: 8g | Sodium: 559mg | Fiber: 7g | Protein: 8g

Easy Falafel Patties

Natural food stores sell a vegan instant falafel mix, but it's not very much work at all to make your own from scratch.

INGREDIENTS | **SERVES 4**

1 (15-ounce) can chickpeas, well drained and rinsed

½ onion, minced

1 tablespoon flour

1 teaspoon cumin

¾ teaspoon garlic powder

¾ teaspoon salt, or to taste

Egg substitute for 1 egg

¼ cup chopped fresh parsley

2 tablespoons chopped fresh cilantro (optional)

1. Preheat oven to 375°F.

2. Place chickpeas in a large bowl and mash with a fork until coarsely mashed, or pulse in a food processor until chopped.

3. Combine chickpeas with onion, flour, cumin, garlic powder, salt, and egg substitute; mash together to combine. Add parsley and cilantro.

4. Shape mixture into 2" balls or 1" thick patties and bake on lightly oiled baking sheet in oven for 15 minutes, or until crisp. Falafel can also be fried in oil for about 5–6 minutes on each side.

PER SERVING Calories: 141 | Fat: 1g | Sodium: 752mg | Fiber: 5g | Protein: 6g

Tofu BBQ Sauce "Steaks"

These chewy tofu "steaks" have a hearty texture and a meaty flavor. Delicious as is, or add it to a sandwich. If you've never cooked tofu before, this is a super-easy foolproof recipe to start with.

INGREDIENTS | SERVES 6

⅓ cup vegan barbecue sauce

¼ cup water

2 teaspoons balsamic vinegar

2 tablespoons soy sauce

1–2 tablespoons hot sauce, or to taste

2 teaspoons sugar

2 blocks (14–16 ounces each) firm or extra-firm tofu, well pressed

½ onion, chopped

2 tablespoons olive oil

1. In a small bowl, whisk together the barbecue sauce, water, vinegar, soy sauce, hot sauce, and sugar until well combined. Set aside.

2. Slice tofu into ¼" thick strips.

3. Sauté onions in oil; carefully add tofu. Fry tofu on both sides until lightly golden brown, about 2 minutes on each side.

4. Reduce heat; add barbecue sauce mixture, stirring to coat tofu well. Cook over medium-low heat until sauce absorbs and thickens, about 5–6 minutes.

PER SERVING Calories: 147 | Fat: 9g | Sodium: 528mg | Fiber: 1g | Protein: 10g

Lentil and Rice Loaf

Made from two of the cheapest ingredients on the planet, this one is a great filler for families on a budget. Serve with mashed potatoes and gravy for an all-American meal. Use poultry seasoning in place of the individual herbs, if you prefer.

INGREDIENTS | SERVES 6

3 cloves garlic

1 large onion, diced

2 tablespoons oil

3½ cups cooked lentils

2¼ cups cooked rice

⅓ cup ketchup plus 3 tablespoons

2 tablespoons flour

Egg replacer for 1 egg

½ teaspoon parsley

½ teaspoon thyme

½ teaspoon oregano

¼ teaspoon sage

¾ teaspoon salt, or to taste

½ teaspoon black pepper

1. Preheat oven to 350°F.

2. Sauté garlic and onions in oil until onions are soft and clear, about 3–4 minutes.

3. In a large bowl, use a fork or a potato masher to mash the lentils until about ⅔ mashed.

4. Add garlic and onions, rice, ⅓ cup ketchup, and flour; combine well. Add egg replacer and remaining seasoning; mash to combine.

5. Gently press the mixture into a lightly greased loaf pan. Drizzle the remaining 3 tablespoons ketchup on top.

6. Bake for 60 minutes. Allow to cool at least 10 minutes before serving, as loaf will firm slightly as it cools.

PER SERVING Calories: 295 | Fat: 5g | Sodium: 528mg | Fiber: 10g | Protein: 13g

Basic Tofu Lasagna

Seasoned tofu takes the place of ricotta cheese in this recipe, and really does look and taste like the real thing. Fresh parsley adds flavor, and with store-bought sauce, it's quick to get in the oven.

INGREDIENTS | SERVES 6

1 block (14–16 ounces) firm tofu
1 (12-ounce) block silken tofu
¼ cup nutritional yeast
1 tablespoon lemon juice
1 tablespoon soy sauce
1 teaspoon garlic powder
2 teaspoons basil
3 tablespoons chopped fresh parsley
1 teaspoon salt, or to taste
4 cups vegan spaghetti sauce
1 (16-ounce) package lasagna noodles, cooked

1. Preheat oven to 350°F.

2. In a large bowl, mash together the firm tofu, silken tofu, nutritional yeast, lemon juice, soy sauce, garlic powder, basil, parsley, and salt until combined and crumbly like ricotta cheese.

3. To assemble the lasagna, spread about ⅔ cup spaghetti sauce on the bottom of a lasagna pan, then add a layer of noodles.

4. Spread about ½ the tofu mixture on top of the noodles, followed by another layer of sauce. Place a second layer of noodles on top, followed by the remaining tofu and more sauce. Finish it off with a third layer of noodles and the rest of the sauce.

5. Cover and bake for 25 minutes.

PER SERVING Calories: 510 | Fat: 10g | Sodium: 1,256mg | Fiber: 8g | Protein: 21g

Easy Pad Thai Noodles

Volumes could be written about Thailand's national dish. It's sweet, sour, spicy, and salty all at once, and filled with as much texture and flavor as the streets of Bangkok themselves.

INGREDIENTS | SERVES 4

1 pound thin rice noodles

¼ cup tahini

¼ cup ketchup

¼ cup soy sauce

2 tablespoons white, rice, or cider vinegar

3 tablespoons lime juice

2 tablespoons sugar

¾ teaspoon crushed red pepper flakes or cayenne

1 block (14–16 ounces) firm or extra-firm tofu, diced small

3 cloves garlic, minced

¼ cup vegetable or safflower oil

4 scallions, chopped

½ teaspoon salt, or to taste

Optional toppings: extra scallions, crushed toasted peanuts, sliced lime

1. Cover the noodles in hot water and set aside to soak until soft, about 5 minutes.

2. Whisk together the tahini, ketchup, soy sauce, vinegar, lime juice, sugar, and pepper flakes.

3. In a large skillet, fry the tofu and garlic in oil until tofu is lightly golden brown, about 8–10 minutes. Add drained noodles, stirring to combine well; fry for 2–3 minutes.

4. Reduce heat to medium; add tahini and ketchup mixture, stirring well to combine. Allow to cook for 3–4 minutes, until well combined and heated through. Add scallions and salt and heat 1 more minute, stirring well.

5. Serve with extra chopped scallions, crushed peanuts, and a lime wedge or two.

PER SERVING Calories: 718 | Fat: 25g | Sodium: 1,401mg | Fiber: 3g | Protein: 11g

Spaghetti with Italian "Meatballs"

These little TVP nuggets are so chewy and addictive, you just might want to make a double batch. If you can't find beef-flavored bouillon, just use what you've got. Don't be tempted to add extra water to the TVP, as it needs to be a little dry for this recipe.

INGREDIENTS | SERVES 6

½ vegetarian beef-flavored bouillon cube (optional)

⅔ cup hot water

⅔ cup TVP

Egg replacer for 2 eggs

½ onion, minced

2 tablespoons ketchup or vegan barbecue sauce

½ teaspoon garlic powder

1 teaspoon basil

1 teaspoon parsley

½ teaspoon sage

½ teaspoon salt, or to taste

½ cup bread crumbs

⅔–¾ cup flour

Oil for pan frying

3 cups prepared vegan spaghetti sauce

1 (12-ounce) package spaghetti noodles, cooked

1. Dissolve bouillon cube in hot water; pour over TVP to reconstitute. Allow to sit for 6–7 minutes. Gently press to remove any excess moisture.

2. In a large bowl, combine the TVP, egg replacer, onion, ketchup, and seasonings until well mixed.

3. Add bread crumbs; combine well. Add flour, a few tablespoons at a time, mixing well to combine, until mixture is sticky and thick. You may need a little more or less than ⅔ cup.

4. Using lightly floured hands, shape into balls 1½"–2" thick.

5. Pan fry "meatballs" in a bit of oil over medium heat, rolling them around in the pan to maintain the shape, until golden brown on all sides, about 10 minutes.

6. Reduce heat to medium low; add spaghetti sauce and heat thoroughly. Serve over noodles.

PER SERVING Calories: 495 | Fat: 9g | Sodium: 850mg | Fiber: 8g | Protein: 18g

Braised Tofu and Veggie Cacciatore

If you'd like a more grown-up Italian dish, use ½ cup white cooking wine in place of ½ cup broth. Serve over pasta or try it with rice, whole grains, or even baked potatoes or polenta.

INGREDIENTS | SERVES 4

½ yellow onion, chopped

½ cup mushrooms, sliced

1 carrot, chopped

3 cloves garlic, minced

2 blocks (14–16 ounces each) firm or extra-firm tofu, chopped into cubes

2 tablespoons olive oil

1½ cups vegetable broth

1 (14-ounce) can diced tomatoes or 3 large fresh tomatoes, diced

1 (6-ounce) can tomato paste

1 bay leaf (optional)

½ teaspoon salt, or to taste

1 teaspoon parsley

1 teaspoon basil

1 teaspoon oregano

1. Sauté the onion, mushrooms, carrot, garlic, and tofu in olive oil for 4–5 minutes, stirring frequently.

2. Reduce heat to medium-low; add vegetable broth, tomatoes, tomato paste, bay leaf, salt, and spices.

3. Cover, and allow to simmer for 20 minutes, stirring occasionally. Remove bay leaf before serving.

PER SERVING Calories: 256 | Fat: 14g | Sodium: 845mg | Fiber: 6g | Protein: 17g

Orange-Glazed "Chicken" Tofu

If you're craving Chinese restaurant–style orange-glazed chicken, try this easy tofu version. It's slightly sweet, slightly salty, and, if you add some crushed red pepper, it'll have a bit of spice as well! Double the sauce and add some veggies for a full meal over rice.

INGREDIENTS | SERVES 3

⅔ cup orange juice

2 tablespoons soy sauce

2 tablespoons rice vinegar

1 tablespoon maple syrup

½ teaspoon red pepper flakes (optional)

2 tablespoons olive oil

1 block (14–16 ounces) firm or extra-firm tofu, well pressed and chopped into 1" cubes

3 cloves garlic, minced

1½ teaspoons cornstarch

2 tablespoons water

1. Whisk together the orange juice, soy sauce, vinegar, maple syrup, and red pepper flakes and set aside.

2. In a large skillet over medium heat, heat the oil; add tofu and garlic. Lightly fry 2–3 minutes.

3. Reduce heat to medium-low; add orange juice mixture. Bring to a very low simmer; cook for 7–8 minutes over low heat.

4. In a small bowl, whisk together the cornstarch and water until cornstarch is dissolved. Add to tofu mixture; stir well to combine.

5. Bring to a simmer; heat for 3–4 minutes, until sauce thickens. Serve over rice or another whole grain, if desired.

PER SERVING Calories: 219 | Fat: 14g | Sodium: 616mg | Fiber: 1g | Protein: 10g

Saucy Kung Pao Tofu

Try adding in a few more Asian ingredients to stretch this recipe—bok choy, water chestnuts, or bamboo shoots—and spoon on top of cooked noodles or plain rice.

INGREDIENTS | SERVES 6

3 tablespoons soy sauce

2 tablespoons rice vinegar or cooking sherry

1 tablespoon sesame oil

2 blocks (14–16 ounces each) firm or extra-firm tofu, chopped into 1" cubes

1 red bell pepper, chopped

1 green bell pepper, chopped

⅔ cup sliced mushrooms

3 cloves garlic, minced

3 small red or green chili peppers, diced small

1 teaspoon red pepper flakes

2 tablespoons oil

1 teaspoon ginger powder

½ cup water or vegetable broth

½ teaspoon sugar

1½ teaspoons cornstarch

2 green onions, chopped

½ cup peanuts

1. In a shallow pan or zip-top bag, whisk together the soy sauce, vinegar, and sesame oil. Add tofu; marinate in the refrigerator for at least 1 hour—the longer the better. Drain tofu, reserving marinade.

2. Sauté bell peppers, mushrooms, garlic, chili peppers, and red pepper flakes in oil for 2–3 minutes; add tofu and heat for another 1–2 minutes, until veggies are almost soft.

3. Reduce heat to medium-low; add marinade, ginger powder, water, sugar, and cornstarch, whisking in the cornstarch to avoid lumps.

4. Heat a few more minutes, stirring constantly, until sauce has almost thickened.

5. Add green onions and peanuts; heat for 1 more minute.

PER SERVING Calories: 535 | Fat: 51g | Sodium: 520mg | Fiber: 3g | Protein: 13g

Sesame Baked Tofu

Baking tofu makes it meaty and chewy, and this is a quick and basic marinade to try if you're new to baking tofu. Serve these marinated tofu strips as an entrée or use as a salad topper or as a meat substitute in a sandwich.

INGREDIENTS | SERVES 6

¼ cup soy sauce

2 tablespoons sesame oil

¾ teaspoon garlic powder

½ teaspoon ginger powder

2 blocks (14–16 ounces each) firm or extra-firm tofu, well pressed

Marinating Tofu

For marinated baked tofu dishes, a zip-top bag can be helpful in getting the tofu well covered with marinade. Place the tofu in the bag, pour the marinade in, seal, and set in the fridge, occasionally turning and lightly shaking to coat all sides of the tofu.

1. Whisk together the soy sauce, sesame oil, garlic, and ginger powder; transfer to a wide, shallow pan.

2. Slice the tofu into ½" thick strips or triangles.

3. Place the tofu in the marinade and coat well. Allow to marinate in the refrigerator for at least 1 hour or overnight.

4. Preheat oven to 400°F.

5. Coat a baking sheet well with nonstick spray or olive oil, or line with foil. Place tofu on sheet.

6. Bake for 20–25 minutes; turn over and bake for another 10–15 minutes, or until done.

PER SERVING Calories: 99 | Fat: 7g | Sodium: 314mg | Fiber: 1g | Protein: 9g

Tofu "Fish" Sticks

Adding seaweed and lemon juice to baked and breaded tofu gives it a "fishy" taste. Crumbled nori sushi sheets would work well too if you can't find kelp or dulse flakes. You could also pan fry these fish sticks in a bit of oil instead of baking, if you prefer.

INGREDIENTS | SERVES 3

½ cup flour

⅓ cup plain or unsweetened soymilk

2 tablespoons lemon juice

1½ cups fine-ground bread crumbs

2 tablespoons kelp or dulse seaweed flakes

1 tablespoon Old Bay seasoning blend

1 teaspoon onion powder

1 block (14–16 ounces) extra-firm tofu, well pressed

Tartar Sauce

To make a simple vegan tartar sauce, combine vegan mayonnaise with sweet pickle relish and a generous squeeze of lemon juice. Or dip your fishy tofu sticks in ketchup or barbecue sauce.

1. Preheat oven to 350°F.

2. Place flour in a shallow bowl or pie tin and set aside.

3. Combine the soymilk and lemon juice in a separate shallow bowl or pie tin.

4. In a third bowl or pie tin, combine the bread crumbs, kelp, Old Bay, and onion powder.

5. Slice tofu into 12, ½" thick strips. Place each strip into the flour mixture to coat well, then dip into the soymilk. Next, place each strip into the bread crumbs, gently patting to coat well.

6. Bake for 15–20 minutes; turn and bake for another 10–15 minutes, or until crispy.

7. Serve with ketchup or vegan tartar sauce.

PER SERVING Calories: 344 | Fat: 8g | Sodium: 1,070mg | Fiber: 4g | Protein: 18g

No Shepherd, No Sheep Pie

Sheepless and shepherdless pie is a hearty vegan entrée!

INGREDIENTS | SERVES 6

1½ cups TVP

1½ cups hot water or vegetable broth

2 tablespoons olive oil

½ onion, chopped

2 cloves garlic, minced

1 large carrot, sliced thin

¾ cup sliced mushrooms

½ cup green peas, fresh or frozen, thawed

½ cup vegetable broth

½ cup soymilk plus 3 tablespoons

1 tablespoon flour

5 medium potatoes, cooked

2 tablespoons vegan margarine

¼ teaspoon rosemary

¼ teaspoon sage

½ teaspoon paprika (optional)

½ teaspoon salt, or to taste

¼ teaspoon black pepper

1. Preheat oven to 350°F.

2. Combine TVP with hot water and allow to sit for 6–7 minutes. Gently drain any excess moisture.

3. In a large skillet, heat oil and sauté onions, garlic, and carrots until onions are soft, about 5 minutes.

4. Add mushrooms, peas, broth, and ½ cup soymilk. Whisk in flour just until sauce thickens; transfer to a casserole dish.

5. Mash together the potatoes, margarine, 3 tablespoons soymilk, rosemary, sage, paprika, salt, and pepper; spread over the vegetables.

6. Bake for 30–35 minutes, or until lightly browned on top.

PER SERVING Calories: 273 | Fat: 4g | Sodium: 373mg | Fiber: 9g | Protein: 17g

Super-Meaty TVP Meatloaf

With a pinkish hue and chewy texture, this meatloaf impersonates the real thing well.
Top with gravy for a Thanksgiving entrée.

INGREDIENTS | SERVES 6

2 cups TVP

1¾ cups hot vegetable broth

1 onion, diced

1 tablespoon oil

¼ cup ketchup

⅓ cup vegan barbecue sauce plus 3 tablespoons

1 cup vital wheat gluten flour

1 cup bread crumbs

1 teaspoon parsley

½ teaspoon sage

½ teaspoon salt, or to taste

¼ teaspoon pepper

1. Combine TVP with broth and allow to sit for 6–7 minutes, until rehydrated. Gently squeeze out any excess moisture.

2. Sauté onion in oil until translucent, about 3–4 minutes.

3. Preheat oven to 400°F.

4. In a large bowl, combine TVP, onions, ketchup, and ⅓ cup barbecue sauce. Add flour, bread crumbs, and spices.

5. Gently press mixture into a lightly greased loaf pan. Drizzle 3 tablespoons of barbecue sauce on top.

6. Bake for 45–50 minutes, until lightly browned. Allow to cool for at least 10 minutes before serving, as loaf will set as it cools.

PER SERVING Calories: 321 | Fat: 4g | Sodium: 967mg | Fiber: 7g | Protein: 33g

Sweet and Sour Tempeh

With maple syrup instead of white sugar, this is a sweet and sour that's slightly less sweet than other versions. There's plenty of sauce, so plan on serving with some plain brown rice or another grain to mop it all up.

INGREDIENTS | SERVES 4

1 cup vegetable broth

2 tablespoons soy sauce

1 (8-ounce) package tempeh, diced into cubes

2 tablespoons vegan barbecue sauce

½ teaspoon ground ginger

2 tablespoons maple syrup

⅓ cup rice vinegar or apple cider vinegar

1 tablespoon cornstarch

1 (15-ounce) can pineapple chunks, drained, juice reserved

2 tablespoons olive oil

1 green bell pepper, chopped

1 red bell pepper, chopped

1 yellow onion, chopped

1. Whisk together the broth and soy sauce and bring to a simmer in a large skillet. Add the tempeh and simmer for 10 minutes. Remove tempeh from the pan; reserve ½ cup broth.

2. In a small bowl, whisk together the barbecue sauce, ginger, maple syrup, vinegar, cornstarch, and juice from pineapples until cornstarch is dissolved. Set aside.

3. Heat olive oil in skillet; add tempeh, bell peppers, and onions. Sauté for 1–2 minutes; add sauce mixture and bring to a simmer.

4. Allow to cook until sauce thickens, about 6–8 minutes. Reduce heat and stir in pineapples. Serve over brown rice or another whole grain.

PER SERVING Calories: 325 | Fat: 13g | Sodium: 795mg | Fiber: 2g | Protein: 13g

CHAPTER 19

Sides: Grains

Coconut Rice

Serve coconut rice as a simple side dish or pair it with spicy Thai and Indian curries or stir-fries.

INGREDIENTS | SERVES 4

1 cup water
1 (14-ounce) can coconut milk
1½ cups white rice, uncooked
⅓ cup coconut flakes
1 teaspoon lime juice
½ teaspoon salt, or to taste

1. In a large pot, combine the water, coconut milk, and rice; bring to a simmer. Cover, and allow to cook 20 minutes, or until rice is done.

2. In a separate skillet, toast the coconut flakes over low heat until lightly golden, about 3 minutes. Gently stir constantly to avoid burning.

3. Combine coconut flakes with cooked rice; stir in lime juice and salt.

PER SERVING Calories: 480 | Fat: 25g | Sodium: 310mg | Fiber: 2g | Protein: 7g

Greek Lemon Rice with Spinach

Greek "spanakorizo" is seasoned with fresh lemon, herbs, and black pepper.
Serve with Lemon Basil Tofu (Chapter 18) for a citrusy meal.

INGREDIENTS | SERVES 4

1 onion, chopped
4 cloves garlic, minced
2 tablespoons olive oil
¾ cup white rice, uncooked
1½ cups water or vegetable broth
1 (8-ounce) can tomato paste
2 bunches fresh spinach, trimmed
2 tablespoons chopped fresh parsley
1 tablespoon chopped fresh mint or dill (optional)
2 tablespoons lemon juice
½ teaspoon salt, or to taste
½ teaspoon fresh ground black pepper

1. Sauté onions and garlic in olive oil for 1–2 minutes; add rice, stirring to lightly toast.

2. Add water; cover, and heat for 10–12 minutes.

3. Add tomato paste, spinach, and parsley. Cover, and cook for another 5 minutes, or until spinach is wilted and rice is cooked.

4. Stir in fresh mint, lemon juice, salt, and pepper.

PER SERVING Calories: 295 | Fat: 8g | Sodium: 488mg | Fiber: 7g | Protein: 10g

Italian Rice Salad

Double this marinated rice salad recipe for a potluck or picnic.

INGREDIENTS | SERVES 4

⅓ cup red wine vinegar

1 tablespoon balsamic vinegar

2 teaspoons Dijon mustard

½ cup olive oil

4 cloves garlic, minced

1 teaspoon basil

⅓ cup chopped fresh parsley

2 cups cooked rice

1 cup green peas, fresh or frozen, thawed

1 carrot, grated

½ cup roasted red peppers, chopped

½ cup green olives, sliced

Salt and pepper, to taste

1. Whisk or shake together the vinegars, mustard, olive oil, garlic, basil, and parsley.

2. In a large bowl, combine rice with remaining ingredients except salt and pepper. Toss with dressing mixture; coat well.

3. Taste, and season with salt and pepper, to taste.

4. Chill for at least 30 minutes before serving to allow flavors to set. Gently toss again just before serving.

PER SERVING Calories: 439 | Fat: 32g | Sodium: 604mg | Fiber: 3g | Protein: 5g

Pineapple Lime Rice

Instead of pineapple, fresh cubed mango would also add a sweet flavor to this simple zesty side.

INGREDIENTS | SERVES 4

2 cups warm, cooked brown or white rice

2 tablespoons vegan margarine

1½ tablespoons lime juice

⅓ cup chopped fresh cilantro

1 (16-ounce) can pineapple tidbits, drained

Dash salt

1. Stir margarine into hot rice until melted and combined.

2. Add remaining ingredients; toss gently to combine. Taste, and add a dash of salt, to taste.

PER SERVING Calories: 222 | Fat: 6g | Sodium: 83mg | Fiber: 2g | Protein: 3g

Sesame Snow Pea Rice Pilaf

The leftovers from this rice pilaf can be enjoyed chilled the next day as a cold rice salad.

INGREDIENTS | SERVES 4

4 cups rice, cooked

2 tablespoons olive oil

1 tablespoon sesame oil

2 tablespoons soy sauce

3 tablespoons apple cider vinegar

1 teaspoon sugar

1 cup snow peas, chopped

¾ cup baby corn, chopped

3 scallions, chopped

2 tablespoons chopped fresh parsley

½ teaspoon sea salt

1. In a large pot over low heat, combine the rice, olive oil, sesame oil, soy sauce, vinegar, and sugar, stirring well to combine.

2. Add snow peas, baby corn, and scallions and heat until warmed through and vegetables are lightly cooked, stirring frequently, so the rice doesn't burn.

3. While still hot, stir in fresh parsley and season well with sea salt.

PER SERVING Calories: 345 | Fat: 11g | Sodium: 839mg | Fiber: 2g | Protein: 7g

Baked Millet Patties

Serve these nutty whole-grain patties topped with Mango Citrus Salsa (Chapter 22), You Are a Goddess Dressing (Chapter 20), or another dressing or sauce.

INGREDIENTS | YIELDS 8 PATTIES

1½ cups cooked millet

½ cup tahini

1 cup bread crumbs

1 teaspoon parsley

¾ teaspoon garlic powder

½ teaspoon onion powder (optional)

⅓ teaspoon salt, or to taste

1. Preheat oven to 350°F.

2. Combine all ingredients together in a bowl; mash to mix well.

3. Use your hands to press firmly into patties, about 1" thick. Place on a baking sheet.

4. Bake for 10–12 minutes on each side.

PER 1 PATTY Calories: 285 | Fat: 10g | Sodium: 214mg | Fiber: 5g | Protein: 9g

Fruited Fall Quinoa

Cranberries and apricots make a sweet combo; add some sage and thyme to give it some more warming flavors and it would make an excellent Thanksgiving side dish.

INGREDIENTS | SERVES 4

1 cup quinoa
2 cups apple juice
1 cup water
½ onion, diced
2 ribs celery, diced
2 tablespoons vegan margarine
½ teaspoon nutmeg
½ teaspoon cinnamon
¼ teaspoon cloves
½ cup dried cranberries
½ cup dried apricots, chopped
1 teaspoon parsley
¼ teaspoon salt, or to taste

1. In a large pot, combine quinoa, apple juice, and water. Cover, and simmer for 15 minutes, or until done.

2. In a large skillet, heat onion and celery in margarine, stirring frequently, until soft, about 5 minutes.

3. Over low heat, combine onions and celery with quinoa; add remaining ingredients, tossing gently to combine. Heat for 3–4 more minutes.

PER SERVING Calories: 360 | Fat: 9g | Sodium: 252mg | Fiber: 6g | Protein: 7g

Lemon Cilantro Couscous

This flavorful couscous is a light and easy side dish, or top it off with a vegetable stew or some stir-fried or roasted veggies for an entrée.

INGREDIENTS | SERVES 4

2 cups vegetable broth
1 cup couscous
⅓ cup lemon juice
½ cup chopped fresh cilantro
¼ teaspoon salt, or to taste

1. Bring broth to a simmer; add couscous. Turn off heat; cover, and let stand for 10 minutes, until soft. Fluff with a fork.

2. Stir in lemon juice and cilantro; season with salt, to taste.

PER SERVING Calories: 174 | Fat: 0g | Sodium: 621mg | Fiber: 2g | Protein: 6g

What Is Couscous?

Couscous isn't technically a whole grain, but rather whole-wheat semolina pasta. But its small size and grainy texture gives it more in common with whole grains than pasta.

Lemon Quinoa Veggie Salad

If you prefer to use fresh veggies, any kind will do.
Steamed broccoli or fresh tomatoes would work well.

INGREDIENTS | SERVES 4

4 cups vegetable broth

1½ cups quinoa

1 cup frozen mixed veggies, thawed

¼ cup lemon juice

¼ cup olive oil

1 teaspoon garlic powder

½ teaspoon salt

¼ teaspoon black pepper

2 tablespoons chopped fresh cilantro or parsley (optional)

1. In a large pot, bring broth to a boil. Add quinoa; cover, and simmer for 15–20 minutes, stirring occasionally, until liquid is absorbed and quinoa is cooked.

2. Add mixed veggies; stir to combine.

3. Remove from heat; combine with remaining ingredients. Serve hot or cold.

PER SERVING Calories: 408 | Fat: 18g | Sodium: 1,261mg | Fiber: 7g | Protein: 11g

Mediterranean Quinoa Pilaf

Inspired by the flavors of the Mediterranean, bring this vibrant whole-grain
dish to a vegan potluck and watch it magically disappear.

INGREDIENTS | SERVES 4

1½ cups quinoa

3 cups vegetable broth

3 tablespoons balsamic vinegar

2 tablespoons olive oil

1 tablespoon lemon juice

⅓ teaspoon salt, or to taste

½ cup sun-dried tomatoes, chopped

½ cup artichoke hearts, chopped

½ cup black or kalamata olives, sliced

1. In a large skillet or saucepan, bring the quinoa and broth to a boil; reduce to a simmer. Cover, and allow quinoa to cook until liquid is absorbed, about 15 minutes. Remove from heat, fluff quinoa with a fork, and allow to stand another 5 minutes.

2. Stir in the vinegar, olive oil, lemon juice, and salt; add remaining ingredients, gently tossing to combine. Serve hot.

PER SERVING Calories: 522 | Fat: 31g | Sodium: 1,168mg | Fiber: 6g | Protein: 11g

Millet and Butternut Squash Casserole

*Slightly sweet, slightly savory, top this millet medley with some
Easy Fried Tofu (Chapter 18) to make it a main meal.*

INGREDIENTS | SERVES 4

1 cup millet

2 cups vegetable broth

1 small butternut squash, peeled, seeded, and chopped

½ cup water

1 teaspoon curry powder

½ cup orange juice

2 tablespoons nutritional yeast

½ teaspoon sea salt, or to taste

1. In a small pot, cook millet in broth until done, about 20–30 minutes.

2. In a separate pan, heat butternut squash in water. Cover, and allow to cook for 10–15 minutes, until squash is almost soft. Remove lid and drain extra water.

3. Combine millet with squash over low heat; add curry and orange juice, stirring to combine well.

4. Heat for 3–4 more minutes; add nutritional yeast and season with salt.

PER SERVING Calories: 242 | Fat: 2g | Sodium: 767mg | Fiber: 6g | Protein: 7g

Orange and Raisin Curried Couscous

*Another whole-grain salad or pilaf that can be served either hot or cold.
Cranberries, currants, or dates may be used instead of raisins.*

INGREDIENTS | SERVES 4

2 cups water or vegetable broth

1½ cups couscous

½ cup orange juice

1 onion, chopped

2 tablespoons olive oil

½ teaspoon coriander powder

1 teaspoon curry powder

2 scallions, chopped

¾ cup golden raisins

¾ cup sliced almonds or pine nuts

1. Bring water to a boil; add couscous and remove from heat.

2. Stir in orange juice; cover, and allow to sit for 15 minutes, until most of the liquid is absorbed and couscous is soft.

3. Heat onion in olive oil for 1–2 minutes; add spices and heat for 1 more minute, until fragrant.

4. Combine couscous with spices; add scallions, raisins, and nuts.

PER SERVING Calories: 520 | Fat: 16g | Sodium: 483mg | Fiber: 7g | Protein: 14g

Mexican Rice with Corn and Peppers

Although Mexican rice is usually just a filling for burritos or served as a side dish, this recipe loads up the veggies, making it hearty enough for a main dish. Use frozen or canned veggies if you need to save time.

INGREDIENTS | SERVES 4

2 cloves garlic, minced

1 cup white rice, uncooked

2 tablespoons olive oil

2 cups vegetable broth

1 cup tomato paste or 4 large tomatoes, puréed

1 green bell pepper, chopped

1 red bell pepper, chopped

Kernels from 1 ear of corn

1 carrot, diced

1 teaspoon chili powder

½ teaspoon cumin

⅓ teaspoon oregano

⅓ teaspoon cayenne pepper, or to taste

⅓ teaspoon salt, or to taste

1. In a large skillet over medium-high heat, add garlic, rice, and olive oil. Toast the rice, stirring frequently, until just golden brown, about 2–3 minutes.

2. Reduce heat; add broth and remaining ingredients.

3. Bring to a simmer; cover, and allow to cook until liquid is absorbed and rice is cooked, about 20–25 minutes, stirring occasionally.

4. Adjust seasonings to taste.

PER SERVING Calories: 342 | Fat: 8g | Sodium: 1,442mg | Fiber: 6g | Protein: 8g

Vegan Burritos

Brown some vegetarian chorizo or mock sausage crumbles, mix with Mexican Rice with Corn and Peppers, and wrap in tortillas, perhaps topped with some shredded vegan cheese, to make vegan burritos.

Spicy Southern Jambalaya

*Make this spicy and smoky Southern rice dish a main meal by adding
in some browned mock sausage or sautéed tofu.*

INGREDIENTS | SERVES 6

2 tablespoons olive oil

1 onion, chopped

1 bell pepper, any color, chopped

1 rib celery, diced

1 (14-ounce) can diced tomatoes, undrained

3 cups water or vegetable broth

2 cups white rice, uncooked

1 bay leaf

1 teaspoon paprika

½ teaspoon thyme

½ teaspoon oregano

½ teaspoon garlic powder

1 cup corn or thawed, frozen mixed diced veggies (optional)

½ teaspoon cayenne or hot Tabasco sauce, to taste

1. In a large skillet or stockpot, heat olive oil. Sauté onion, bell pepper, and celery until almost soft, about 3 minutes.

2. Reduce heat and add remaining ingredients except veggies and cayenne; cover. Bring to a low simmer; cook for 20 minutes, until rice is done, stirring occasionally.

3. Add veggies and cayenne; cook just until heated through, about 3 minutes. Adjust seasonings to taste. Remove bay leaf before serving.

PER SERVING Calories: 304 | Fat: 7g | Sodium: 100mg | Fiber: 4g | Protein: 7g

Got Leftovers?

Heat up some refried beans and wrap up your leftover jambalaya in tortillas with some salsa and shredded lettuce to make New Orleans-style vegetable burritos!

Sun-Dried Tomato Risotto with Spinach and Pine Nuts

*The tomatoes carry the flavor in this easy risotto—no butter, cheese, or wine is needed.
But if you're a gourmand who keeps truffle, hazelnut, pine nut, or another gourmet oil on hand,
now's the time to use it, instead of the margarine.*

INGREDIENTS | SERVES 4

1 yellow onion, diced

4 cloves garlic, minced

2 tablespoons olive oil

1½ cups arborio rice, uncooked

5–6 cups vegetable broth

⅔ cup rehydrated sun-dried tomatoes, sliced

½ cup fresh spinach

1 tablespoon chopped fresh basil (optional)

2 tablespoons vegan margarine (optional)

2 tablespoons nutritional yeast

Salt and pepper, to taste

¼ cup pine nuts

1. Heat onion and garlic in olive oil until just soft, about 2–3 minutes. Add rice; toast for 1 minute, stirring constantly.

2. Add ¾ cup broth; stir to combine. When most of the liquid has been absorbed, add another ½ cup, stirring constantly. Continue adding liquid ½ cup at a time until rice is cooked, about 20 minutes.

3. Add another ½ cup broth, tomatoes, spinach, and basil; reduce heat to low. Stir to combine well. Heat for 3–4 minutes, until tomatoes are soft and spinach is wilted.

4. Stir in margarine and nutritional yeast. Taste, then season with salt and pepper, to taste.

5. Allow to cool slightly, then top with pine nuts. Risotto will thicken a bit as it cools.

PER SERVING Calories: 441 | Fat: 13g | Sodium: 1,322mg | Fiber: 4g | Protein: 8g

"Cheesy" Broccoli and Rice Casserole

If you're substituting frozen broccoli, there's no need to cook it first,
just thaw and use about 1¼ cups.

INGREDIENTS | SERVES 4

1 head broccoli, chopped small
1 onion, chopped
4 cloves garlic, minced
2 tablespoons olive oil
2 tablespoons flour
2 cups unsweetened soymilk
½ cup vegetable broth
2 tablespoons nutritional yeast
1 tablespoon vegan margarine
¼ teaspoon nutmeg
¼ teaspoon mustard powder
½ teaspoon salt
3½ cups cooked rice
⅔ cup bread crumbs or crushed vegan crackers

1. Preheat oven to 325°F.

2. Steam or microwave broccoli until just barely soft; do not overcook.

3. Sauté onions and garlic in olive oil until soft, about 3–4 minutes. Reduce heat and add flour, stirring continuously to combine.

4. Add soymilk and vegetable broth and heat, stirring, until thickened. Remove from heat and stir in nutritional yeast, margarine, nutmeg, mustard powder, and salt.

5. Combine sauce, steamed broccoli, and cooked rice and transfer to a large casserole or baking dish. Sprinkle the top with bread crumbs or vegan crackers.

6. Cover and bake for 25 minutes. Uncover and cook for another 10 minutes.

PER SERVING Calories: 477 | Fat: 14g | Sodium: 401mg | Fiber: 7g | Protein: 16g

Barley and Mushroom Pilaf

An earthy-flavored pilaf with mushrooms and nutty toasted barley.
This one will really stick to your ribs!

INGREDIENTS | SERVES 4

1 cup sliced porcini mushrooms

1 cup sliced shiitake mushrooms

2 ribs celery, diced

½ onion, chopped

3 tablespoons vegan margarine or olive oil, divided

1¼ cups barley

3¾ cups vegetable broth

1 bay leaf

¼ teaspoon sage

½ teaspoon parsley

½ teaspoon thyme

1. In a large skillet or stock pot, sauté mushrooms, celery, and onion in 2 tablespoons margarine until almost soft, about 2–3 minutes.

2. Add barley and remaining 1 tablespoon of margarine; allow to toast for 1–2 minutes, stirring frequently.

3. When barley starts to turn brown, add broth and seasonings.

4. Bring to a simmer; cover, and allow to cook for 20–25 minutes, stirring occasionally, until liquid is absorbed and barley is cooked. Remove bay leaf before serving.

PER SERVING Calories: 323 | Fat: 9g | Sodium: 1,025mg | Fiber: 11g | Protein: 8g

Cooking Barley

Be sure you pick up either pearl or quick-cooking barley, and not the hulled variety, which takes ages to cook. Pearl barley is done in 20–25 minutes, and quick-cooking barley is done in about 10, so adjust the cooking times as needed. Barley can also be cooked in your rice steamer with about 2½ cups liquid for each cup of barley.

Bulgur Wheat Tabbouleh Salad with Tomatoes

Though you'll need to adjust the cooking time, of course, you can try this tabbouleh recipe with just about any whole grain. Bulgur wheat is traditional, but quinoa, millet, or amaranth would also work.

INGREDIENTS | SERVES 4

1¼ cups boiling water or vegetable broth

1 cup bulgur wheat

3 tablespoons olive oil

¼ cup lemon juice

1 teaspoon garlic powder

½ teaspoon salt

½ teaspoon pepper

3 scallions, chopped

½ cup chopped fresh mint

½ cup chopped fresh parsley

1 (15-ounce) can chickpeas, drained (optional)

3 large tomatoes, diced

1. Pour boiling water over bulgur wheat. Cover; allow to sit for 30 minutes, or until bulgur wheat is soft.

2. Toss bulgur wheat with olive oil, lemon juice, garlic powder, and salt, stirring well to coat. Combine with remaining ingredients, adding in tomatoes last.

3. Allow to chill for at least 1 hour before serving.

PER SERVING Calories: 252 | Fat: 11g | Sodium: 315mg | Fiber: 10g | Protein: 7g

Leftover Tabbouleh Sandwiches

Spread a slice of bread or a tortilla with some hummus, then layer leftover tabbouleh, sweet pickle relish, thinly sliced cucumbers, and some lettuce to make a quick sandwich or wrap for lunch.

Confetti "Rice" with TVP

If the kids like Mexican rice, try this whole-grain version with barley and TVP.

INGREDIENTS | SERVES 6

2 tablespoons olive oil

1 onion, chopped

2 cloves garlic, minced

1 cup barley

1 (15-ounce) can diced tomatoes

2 cups vegetable broth

1 teaspoon chili powder

½ teaspoon cumin

¾ cup TVP

1 cup hot water or vegetable broth

1 tablespoon soy sauce

1 cup thawed, frozen veggie mix (peas, corn, and carrots)

1 teaspoon parsley

½ teaspoon salt, or to taste

1. In a large skillet, heat the olive oil. Add the onion and garlic; sauté for 1–2 minutes. Add barley; toast for 1 minute, stirring constantly.

2. Add tomatoes including liquid, broth, chili powder, and cumin. Cook until barley is almost soft, about 15 minutes.

3. While barley is cooking, combine TVP with hot water and soy sauce; allow to sit for 8–10 minutes, until TVP is rehydrated. Drain any excess liquid.

4. When barley is almost done cooking, add rehydrated TVP, veggies, parsley, and salt. Heat for another 5 minutes, or until done.

PER SERVING Calories: 258 | Fat: 5g | Sodium: 628mg | Fiber: 11g | Protein: 12g

Turn It Into Tacos

Use this "meaty" Mexican "rice" as a base for burritos or crunchy tacos instead of meat, along with some shredded lettuce, vegan cheese, and nondairy sour cream or serve alongside some cooked beans for a healthy Mexican meal.

Quinoa and Fresh Herb Stuffing

Substitute dried herbs if you have to, but fresh is best in this untraditional stuffing recipe.

INGREDIENTS | SERVES 6

1 yellow onion, chopped

2 ribs celery, diced

¼ cup vegan margarine

1 teaspoon chopped fresh rosemary

2 teaspoons chopped fresh marjoram

1½ tablespoons chopped fresh thyme

1 tablespoon chopped fresh sage

6 slices dried bread, cubed

1¼ cup vegetable broth

2 cups cooked quinoa

¾ teaspoon salt, or to taste

½ teaspoon pepper

Stuffed-Up Stuffing

Stuffing works best with dried bread to better absorb all that flavor and moisture. Leave your bread out for a couple days, or lightly toast in a 275°F oven for 20 minutes on each side. For a more textured stuffing, add in ¾ cup chopped dried apricots, ¾ cup chopped nuts (walnuts, cashews, or pecans), or sauté some mushrooms or a grated carrot along with the onions and celery.

1. Preheat oven to 400°F.

2. Sauté onion and celery in margarine until soft, about 6–8 minutes. Add fresh herbs; heat for another minute, just until fragrant.

3. Remove from heat; pour into a casserole dish.

4. Add bread; combine well. Add vegetable broth to moisten bread; you may need a bit more or less than 1¼ cups.

5. Add cooked quinoa, salt, and pepper; combine well.

6. Cover; bake for 30 minutes.

PER SERVING Calories: 220 | Fat: 10g | Sodium: 739mg | Fiber: 3g | Protein: 5g

Summer Squash and Barley Risotto

A smooth and saucy risotto with barley instead of rice. Fresh asparagus instead of squash would also be lovely in this untraditional risotto. Top it off with some vegan Parmesan cheese, if you happen to have some on hand.

INGREDIENTS | SERVES 4

4 cloves garlic, minced
½ onion, diced
1 zucchini, chopped
1 yellow squash, chopped
2 tablespoons olive oil
1 cup pearled barley
3–4 cups vegetable broth
2 tablespoons chopped fresh basil
2 tablespoons nutritional yeast
2 tablespoons vegan margarine
Salt and pepper, to taste

1. Sauté garlic, onions, zucchini, and yellow squash in olive oil until soft, about 3–4 minutes. Add barley; heat for 1 minute, stirring to coat well with oil and to prevent burning.

2. Add 1 cup broth; bring to a simmer. Cover; allow to cook for a few minutes, until broth is almost absorbed.

3. Add another cup of broth; continue cooking until barley is soft, about 20–25 minutes, adding more broth as needed.

4. When barley is done, add an additional ¼ cup broth and basil; stir well to combine just until heated through.

5. Stir in yeast and margarine; season generously with salt and pepper, to taste.

PER SERVING Calories: 323 | Fat: 13g | Sodium: 797mg | Fiber: 9g | Protein: 7g

CHAPTER 20

Sides: Salads and Vegetables

Carrot and Date Salad

*If you're used to carrot and raisin salads with pineapple and drowning in mayonnaise,
this lighter version with tahini, dates, and mandarin oranges will be a welcome change.*

INGREDIENTS | SERVES 4

⅓ cup tahini

1 tablespoon olive oil

2 tablespoons agave nectar or 2 teaspoons sugar

3 tablespoons lemon juice

¼ teaspoon salt

4 large carrots, grated

½ cup chopped dates

3 Satsuma or mandarin oranges, sectioned

⅓ cup coconut flakes (optional)

1. In a small bowl, whisk together the tahini, olive oil, agave nectar, lemon juice, and salt.

2. Place grated carrots in a large bowl; toss well with tahini mixture.

3. Add dates, oranges, and coconut flakes; combine well.

4. Allow to sit for at least 1 hour before serving to soften carrots and dates. Toss again before serving.

PER SERVING Calories: 307 | Fat: 15g | Sodium: 220mg | Fiber: 7g | Protein: 5g

Edamame Salad

If you can't find shelled edamame, try this recipe with lima beans instead.

INGREDIENTS | SERVES 4

2 cups frozen shelled edamame, thawed and drained

1 red or yellow bell pepper, diced

¾ cup corn kernels, fresh or frozen and thawed

3 tablespoons chopped fresh cilantro (optional)

3 tablespoons olive oil

2 tablespoons red wine vinegar

1 teaspoon soy sauce

1 teaspoon chili powder

2 teaspoons lemon or lime juice

Salt and pepper, to taste

1. In a large bowl, combine edamame, bell pepper, corn, and cilantro.

2. Whisk together the olive oil, vinegar, soy sauce, chili powder, and lemon juice; combine with the edamame. Add salt and pepper, to taste.

3. Chill for at least 1 hour before serving.

PER SERVING Calories: 246 | Fat: 16g | Sodium: 133mg | Fiber: 9g | Protein: 10g

Italian White Bean and Fresh Herb Salad

Don't let the simplicity of this bean salad fool you! The fresh herbs marinate the beans to flavorful perfection, so there's no need to add anything else!

INGREDIENTS | SERVES 4

2 (14.5-ounce) cans cannellini or great northern beans, drained and rinsed

2 ribs celery, diced

¼ cup chopped fresh parsley

¼ cup chopped fresh basil

3 tablespoons olive oil

3 large tomatoes, chopped

½ cup sliced black olives

2 tablespoons lemon juice

Salt and pepper, to taste

¼ teaspoon crushed red pepper flakes (optional)

1. In a large skillet, combine the beans, celery, parsley, and basil with olive oil. Heat, stirring frequently, over low heat for 3 minutes, until herbs are softened but not cooked.

2. Remove from heat; stir in remaining ingredients, gently tossing to combine. Chill for at least 1 hour before serving.

PER SERVING Calories: 377 | Fat: 14g | Sodium: 279mg | Fiber: 12g | Protein: 16g

Kidney Bean and Chickpea Salad

This marinated two-bean salad is perfect for summer picnics or as a side for outdoor barbecues or potlucks.

INGREDIENTS | SERVES 6

¼ cup olive oil

¼ cup red wine vinegar

½ teaspoon paprika

2 tablespoons lemon juice

1 (14-ounce) can chickpeas, drained and rinsed

1 (14-ounce) can kidney beans, drained and rinsed

½ cup sliced black olives

1 (8-ounce) can corn, drained

½ red onion, chopped

1 tablespoon chopped fresh parsley

Salt and pepper, to taste

1. Whisk together olive oil, vinegar, paprika, and lemon juice.

2. In a large bowl, combine the chickpeas, beans, olives, corn, onion, and parsley. Pour the dressing over the bean mixture; toss well to combine.

3. Season generously with salt and pepper, to taste.

4. Chill for at least 1 hour before serving to allow flavors to mingle.

PER SERVING Calories: 252 | Fat: 12g | Sodium: 569mg | Fiber: 8g | Protein: 7g

Lemon-Cumin Potato Salad

A mayonnaise-free potato salad with exotic flavors, this one is delicious either hot or cold.

INGREDIENTS | SERVES 4

1 small yellow onion, diced

2 tablespoons olive oil

1½ teaspoons cumin

4 large cooked potatoes, chopped

3 tablespoons lemon juice

2 teaspoons Dijon mustard

1 scallion, chopped

¼ teaspoon cayenne pepper

2 tablespoons chopped fresh cilantro (optional)

1. In a skillet over medium heat, add the olive oil. Once the oil is warm, add onions and cook until soft, about 5 minutes.

2. Add cumin and potatoes; cook for just 1 minute, stirring well to combine. Remove from heat.

3. Whisk together the lemon juice and Dijon mustard; pour over potatoes, tossing gently to coat.

4. Add scallions, cayenne pepper, and cilantro; combine well.

5. Chill before serving.

PER SERVING Calories: 360 | Fat: 7g | Sodium: 53mg | Fiber: 9g | Protein: 8g

No-Mayo Apple Coleslaw

There's nothing wrong with grabbing a store-bought, preshredded coleslaw mix from the produce section to make this vegan salad, just double the dressing if you find it's not enough.

INGREDIENTS | SERVES 4

1 head cabbage, shredded

1 apple, diced small

1 (15-ounce) can pineapple, drained, 2 tablespoons juice reserved

1 tablespoon apple cider vinegar

2 tablespoons olive oil

1 tablespoon tahini

2 tablespoons agave nectar *or* 1 teaspoon sugar

2 tablespoons sunflower seeds (optional)

1. In a large bowl, combine the cabbage, apple, and pineapple.

2. In a separate small bowl, whisk together 2 tablespoons of the pineapple juice with the cider vinegar, olive oil, and tahini. Pour over cabbage and apples; toss gently to coat.

3. Drizzle with agave nectar; toss to coat.

4. Chill for at least 30 minutes before serving. Toss with sunflower seeds.

PER SERVING Calories: 196 | Fat: 2g | Sodium: 47mg | Fiber: 8g | Protein: 4g

Spicy Sweet Cucumber Salad

Japanese cucumber salad is cool and refreshing, but with a bit of spice.
Enjoy it as a healthy afternoon snack or as a fresh accompaniment to take-out.

INGREDIENTS | SERVES 2

2 cucumbers, thinly sliced

¾ teaspoon salt

¼ cup rice wine vinegar

1 teaspoon sugar *or* 1 tablespoon agave nectar

1 teaspoon sesame oil

¼ teaspoon red pepper flakes

½ onion, thinly sliced

1. In a large shallow container or baking sheet, spread the cucumbers in a single layer; sprinkle with salt. Allow to sit at least 10 minutes.

2. Drain any excess water from the cucumbers.

3. Whisk together the rice wine vinegar, sugar, oil, and red pepper flakes.

4. Pour dressing over the cucumbers; add onions, and toss gently.

5. Allow to sit at least 10 minutes before serving to allow flavors to mingle.

PER SERVING Calories: 90 | Fat: 3g | Sodium: 880mg | Fiber: 2g | Protein: 2g

Dairy-Free Ranch Dressing

An all-American creamy homemade ranch dressing, without the buttermilk.
Get those baby carrots ready to dip!

INGREDIENTS | YIELDS 1 CUP

1 (12-ounce) block silken tofu

2½ tablespoons lemon juice

1 teaspoon prepared yellow mustard

1½ teaspoons apple cider or white vinegar

1 teaspoon sugar

½ teaspoon salt

⅓ cup canola or safflower oil

¼ cup soymilk

1 teaspoon Dijon mustard

1¾ teaspoon onion powder

¾ teaspoon garlic powder

1 tablespoon minced fresh chives

1. In a food processor, process tofu, lemon juice, mustard, vinegar, sugar, and salt until smooth.

2. On high speed, slowly incorporate the oil just a few drops at a time, until smooth and creamy.

3. Whisk or blend in remaining ingredients except chives until smooth.

4. Stir in chives until well combined.

PER TABLESPOON Calories: 57 | Fat: 5g | Sodium: 83mg | Fiber: 0g | Protein: 1g

Thai Orange Peanut Dressing

A sweet and spicy take on traditional Thai and Indonesian peanut and satay sauce.
Add a bit less liquid to use this salad dressing as a dip for veggies.

INGREDIENTS | YIELDS ¾ CUP

¼ cup peanut butter, room temperature

¼ cup orange juice

2 tablespoons soy sauce

2 tablespoons rice vinegar

2 tablespoons water

½ teaspoon garlic powder

½ teaspoon sugar

¼ teaspoon crushed red chili flakes
(optional)

Whisk together all ingredients until smooth and creamy, adding more or less liquid to achieve desired consistency.

PER TABLESPOON Calories: 36 | Fat: 3g | Sodium: 176mg | Fiber: 0g | Protein: 1g

You Are a Goddess Dressing

Turn this zesty salad dressing into a dip for veggies or a sandwich spread
by reducing the amount of liquids.

INGREDIENTS | YIELDS 1½ CUPS

⅔ cup tahini

¼ cup apple cider vinegar

⅓ cup soy sauce

2 teaspoons lemon juice

1 clove garlic

¾ teaspoon sugar (optional)

⅓ cup olive oil

1. In a blender or food processor, process all the ingredients except olive oil until blended.

2. With the blender or food processor on high speed, slowly add in the olive oil, blending for a full minute to allow the oil to emulsify.

3. Chill in the refrigerator for at least 10 minutes before serving; dressing will thicken as it chills.

PER TABLESPOON Calories: 70 | Fat: 7g | Sodium: 208mg | Fiber: 1g | Protein: 1g

In Search of Tahini

Tahini is a sesame seed paste native to Middle Eastern cuisine with a thinner consistency and milder flavor than peanut butter. You'll find a jarred or canned version in the ethnic foods aisle of large grocery stores.

Baked Sweet Potato Fries

Brown sugar adds a sweet touch to these yummy sweet potato fries. If you like your fries with a kick, add some crushed red pepper flakes or a dash of cayenne pepper to the mix.

INGREDIENTS | SERVES 3

2 large sweet potatoes, sliced into fries
2 tablespoons olive oil
¼ teaspoon garlic powder
½ teaspoon paprika
½ teaspoon brown sugar
½ teaspoon chili powder
¼ teaspoon salt

1. Preheat oven to 400°F.

2. Spread sweet potatoes on a large baking sheet; drizzle with olive oil, tossing gently to coat.

3. In a small bowl, combine remaining ingredients. Sprinkle over potatoes; coat evenly and toss as needed.

4. Bake in oven for 10 minutes, turning once. Taste, and add more salt, to taste.

PER SERVING Calories: 203 | Fat: 9g | Sodium: 270mg | Fiber: 4g | Protein: 2g

Cajun Collard Greens

Collard greens are a great choice to add calcium and iron to your diet. Add some zesty Cajun seasonings to make them even more appealing.

INGREDIENTS | SERVES 4

1 onion, diced
3 cloves garlic, minced
1 pound collard greens, chopped
2 tablespoons olive oil
¾ cup water or vegetable broth
1 (14-ounce) can diced tomatoes, drained
1½ teaspoons Cajun seasoning
½ teaspoon hot sauce, or to taste
¼ teaspoon salt, or to taste

1. In a large skillet, sauté onions, garlic, and collard greens in olive oil for 3–5 minutes, until onions are soft.

2. Add water, tomatoes, and Cajun seasoning. Bring to a simmer; cover, and allow to cook for 20 minutes, or until greens are soft, stirring occasionally.

3. Remove lid, and stir in hot sauce and salt; cook, uncovered, for 1–2 minutes, to allow excess moisture to evaporate.

PER SERVING Calories: 125 | Fat: 7g | Sodium: 517mg | Fiber: 6g | Protein: 4g

Creamed Spinach and Mushrooms

The combination of greens and nutritional yeast is simply delicious and provides an excellent jolt of nutrients that vegans need. Don't forget that spinach will shrink when cooked, so use lots!

INGREDIENTS | SERVES 4

½ onion, diced
2 cloves garlic, minced
1½ cups sliced mushrooms
2 tablespoons olive oil
1 tablespoon flour
2 bunches fresh spinach, trimmed
1 cup original or unsweetened soymilk
1 tablespoon vegan margarine
¼ teaspoon nutmeg (optional)
2 tablespoons nutritional yeast (optional)
Salt and pepper, to taste

1. Sauté onion, garlic, and mushrooms in olive oil for 3–4 minutes. Add flour; heat, stirring constantly, for 1 minute.

2. Reduce heat to medium low; add spinach and soymilk. Cook uncovered for 8–10 minutes, until spinach is soft and liquid has reduced.

3. Stir in remaining ingredients; season with salt and pepper, to taste.

PER SERVING Calories: 169 | Fat: 11g | Sodium: 206mg | Fiber: 5g | Protein: 8g

Lemon-Mint New Potatoes

Potatoes are an easy standby side that goes with just about any entrée, and this version with fresh mint adds a twist to the usual herb-roasted version.

INGREDIENTS | SERVES 4

10–12 small new potatoes, chopped
4 cloves garlic, minced
1 tablespoon olive oil
¼ cup chopped mint
Salt and pepper, to taste
2 teaspoons lemon juice

1. Preheat oven to 350°F. Line or lightly grease a baking sheet.

2. In a large bowl, toss together the potatoes, garlic, olive oil, and mint, coating potatoes well.

3. Arrange potatoes in a single layer on a baking sheet; roast for 45 minutes.

4. Season with salt and pepper and drizzle with lemon juice just before serving.

PER SERVING Calories: 330 | Fat: 4g | Sodium: 28mg | Fiber: 11g | Protein: 8g

Got Leftovers?

Make a double batch to have planned-overs. Turn this into a Greek-inspired potato salad for lunch the next day. Cool the potatoes, then combine with ¼ cup vegan yogurt, green peas, diced red onions or celery, and some extra fresh mint for garnish and flavor.

Summer Squash Sauté

Green zucchini and yellow squash absorb flavors like magic, though little enhancement is needed with their fresh natural flavor. Toss these veggies with some cooked orzo or linguini to make it a main dish.

INGREDIENTS | SERVES 2

1 onion, chopped

2 cloves garlic, minced

2 tablespoons olive oil

2 zucchini, sliced into coins

2 yellow squash, sliced thin

1 large tomato, diced

2 teaspoons Italian seasoning

1 tablespoon nutritional yeast

2 teaspoons hot chili sauce (optional)

1. In a large skillet over medium heat, sauté onions and garlic in olive oil for 1–2 minutes.

2. Add zucchini, squash, and tomato. Heat, stirring frequently, for 4–5 minutes, until squash is soft.

3. Season with Italian seasoning; heat for 1 minute.

4. Stir in yeast and hot sauce.

PER SERVING Calories: 205 | Fat: 14g | Sodium: 28mg | Fiber: 5g | Protein: 5g

Gingered Bok Choy and Tofu Stir-Fry

Dark, leafy bok choy is a highly nutritious vegetable that can be found in well-stocked groceries. Keep an eye out for light-green baby bok choy, which is a bit more tender but carry a similar flavor.

INGREDIENTS | SERVES 3

3 tablespoons soy sauce

2 tablespoons lemon or lime juice

1 tablespoon fresh ginger, minced

1 block (14–16 ounces) firm or extra-firm tofu, well pressed

2 tablespoons olive oil

1 head bok choy or 3–4 small baby bok choys, chopped

½ teaspoon sugar

½ teaspoon sesame oil

1. In a shallow pan, whisk together soy sauce, lemon juice, and ginger.

2. Cut tofu into cubes; marinate in the refrigerator for at least 1 hour. Drain, reserving marinade.

3. In a large skillet or wok, sauté tofu in olive oil for 3–4 minutes.

4. Carefully add reserved marinade, bok choy, and sugar; stir well to combine.

5. Cook, stirring, for 3–4 more minutes.

6. Drizzle with sesame oil. Serve over rice.

PER SERVING Calories: 213 | Fat: 15g | Sodium: 1,097mg | Fiber: 4g | Protein: 14g

Maple-Glazed Roasted Veggies

These easy roasted veggies make an excellent holiday side dish. The vegetables can be roasted in advance and reheated with the glaze to save on time, if needed. If parsnips are too earthy for you, substitute one large potato.

INGREDIENTS | SERVES 4

3 carrots, peeled and chopped

2 small parsnips, peeled and chopped

2 sweet potatoes, chopped

2 tablespoons olive oil

Salt and pepper, to taste

⅓ cup maple syrup

2 tablespoons Dijon mustard

1 tablespoon balsamic vinegar

½ teaspoon hot sauce

1. Preheat oven to 400°F.

2. On a large baking sheet, spread out carrots, parsnips, and sweet potatoes.

3. Drizzle with olive oil and season to taste with salt and pepper. Roast for 40 minutes, tossing once.

4. In a small bowl, whisk together syrup, mustard, vinegar, and hot sauce.

5. Transfer the roasted vegetables to a large bowl; toss well with the maple mixture. Add salt and pepper, to taste.

PER SERVING Calories: 231 | Fat: 7g | Sodium: 158mg | Fiber: 5g | Protein: 5g

Orange and Ginger Mixed-Veggie Stir-Fry

Rice vinegar can be substituted for the apple cider vinegar, if you prefer. As with most stir-fry recipes, the vegetables are merely a suggestion; use your favorites or whatever looks like it's been sitting too long in your crisper.

INGREDIENTS | SERVES 4

3 tablespoons orange juice

1 tablespoon apple cider vinegar

2 tablespoons soy sauce

2 tablespoons water

1 tablespoon maple syrup

1 teaspoon powdered ginger

2 cloves garlic, minced

2 tablespoons oil

1 bunch broccoli, chopped

½ cup sliced mushrooms

½ cup snap peas, chopped

1 carrot, sliced

1 cup chopped cabbage or bok choy

1. Whisk together the orange juice, vinegar, soy sauce, water, maple syrup, and ginger.

2. Heat oil in a large skillet, add garlic and cook for 1–2 minutes; add veggies. Allow to cook over high heat, stirring frequently, for 2–3 minutes, until just starting to get tender.

3. Add sauce and reduce heat; simmer, stirring frequently, for another 3–4 minutes, or until veggies are cooked.

PER SERVING Calories: 117 | Fat: 3g | Sodium: 518mg | Fiber: 6g | Protein: 6g

Roasted-Garlic Mashed Potatoes

In the absence of milk and butter, load up your mashed potatoes with roasted garlic for a flavor blast.

INGREDIENTS | SERVES 4

1 whole head garlic
2 tablespoons olive oil
6 potatoes, cooked
¼ cup vegan margarine
½ cup soy creamer or soymilk
Salt and pepper, to taste

1. Heat oven to 400°F.

2. Remove outer layer of skin from garlic head. Drizzle generously with olive oil, wrap in aluminum foil, and place on a baking sheet. Roast in oven for 30 minutes.

3. Gently press cloves out of the skins; mash smooth with a fork.

4. Using a mixer or a potato masher, combine garlic with potatoes, margarine, and creamer until smooth.

5. Season to taste with salt and pepper.

PER SERVING Calories: 367 | Fat: 14g | Sodium: 199mg | Fiber: 8g | Protein: 6g

Sweet Pineapple Cabbage Stir-Fry

Toss in a can of pineapple the last minute or 2 to just about any stir-fry recipe for a sweet treat.

INGREDIENTS | SERVES 6

1 (15-ounce) can diced pineapple
2 tablespoons red wine vinegar
1 tablespoon soy sauce
1 tablespoon brown sugar
2 teaspoons cornstarch
¼ teaspoon crushed red pepper flakes
2 cloves garlic, minced
1 onion, chopped
2 tablespoons olive oil
1 head broccoli, chopped
1 head Napa cabbage or ½ head green cabbage, chopped
1 batch Easy Fried Tofu (Chapter 18, optional)

1. Drain pineapple, reserving juice. In a medium bowl, whisk together pineapple juice, vinegar, soy sauce, brown sugar, cornstarch, and red pepper flakes.

2. In a large skillet heat olive oil, add garlic and onion and cook just until soft, about 3–4 minutes.

3. Add broccoli, pineapple, and cabbage. Stir quickly to combine; cook for 1 minute.

4. Reduce heat to medium; add pineapple juice mixture. Bring to a slow simmer; heat just until mixture has thickened, about 3–5 minutes, stirring frequently.

5. Stir in fried tofu. Serve over rice or whole grains.

PER SERVING Calories: 288 | Fat: 17g | Sodium: 357mg | Fiber: 5g | Protein: 13g

CHAPTER 21

Soups and Stews

"Chicken" Noodle Soup

If you think you're getting a cold, this vegan soup is even more comforting and delicious than its nonvegan counterpart.

INGREDIENTS | SERVES 6

6 cups vegetable broth

1 carrot, diced

2 ribs celery, diced

1 onion, chopped

½ cup TVP

2 bay leaves

1½ teaspoons Italian seasonings

Salt and pepper, to taste

1 cup vegan noodles or small pasta

1. Combine all ingredients in a large soup or stockpot.

2. Cover and simmer for 15–20 minutes.

PER SERVING Calories: 123 | Fat: 0g | Sodium: 960mg | Fiber: 3g | Protein: 7g

Black Bean and Butternut Squash Chili

Squash is an excellent addition to vegetarian chili in this Southwestern-style dish.

INGREDIENTS | SERVES 6

1 onion, chopped

3 cloves garlic, minced

2 tablespoons olive oil

1 medium butternut squash, peeled and chopped into chunks

2 (15-ounce) cans black beans, drained and rinsed

1 (28-ounce) can stewed or diced tomatoes, undrained

¾ cup water or vegetable broth

1 tablespoon chili powder

1 teaspoon cumin

¼ teaspoon cayenne pepper, or to taste

½ teaspoon salt, or to taste

2 tablespoons chopped fresh cilantro (optional)

1. In a large stockpot, sauté onion and garlic in oil until soft, about 4 minutes.

2. Reduce heat; add remaining ingredients except cilantro.

3. Cover and simmer for 25 minutes.

4. Uncover and simmer another 5 minutes. Top with fresh cilantro just before serving.

PER SERVING Calories: 303 | Fat: 6g | Sodium: 832mg | Fiber: 17g | Protein: 18g

Shiitake and Garlic Broth

Shiitake mushrooms transform ordinary broth into a rich stock with a deep flavor.

INGREDIENTS | YIELDS 6 CUPS BROTH

⅓ cup dried shiitake mushrooms

6 cups water

2 cloves garlic, smashed

1 bay leaf

½ teaspoon thyme

½ onion, chopped

1. In a large soup or stockpot, combine all ingredients; bring to a slow simmer.

2. Cover and allow to cook for at least 30–40 minutes.

3. Strain before using.

PER 1 CUP Calories: 8 | Fat: 0g | Sodium: 5mg | Fiber: 0g | Protein: 0g

Vegetarian Dashi

To turn this into a Japanese dashi stock for miso and noodle soups, omit the bay leaf and thyme and add a generous amount of seaweed, preferably kombu, if you can find it!

African Peanut and Greens Soup

Cut back on the red pepper flakes to make this soup for kids, or reduce the liquids to turn it into a thick and chunky curry to pour over rice. Although the ingredients are all familiar, this is definitely not a boring meal!

INGREDIENTS | SERVES 4

1 onion, diced

3 tomatoes, chopped

2 tablespoons olive oil

2 cups vegetable broth

1 cup coconut milk

⅓ cup peanut butter

1 (15-ounce) can chickpeas, drained and rinsed

½ teaspoon salt, or to taste

1 teaspoon curry powder

1 teaspoon sugar

⅓ teaspoon red pepper flakes

1 bunch fresh spinach, stemmed

1. Sauté the onions and tomatoes in olive oil until onions are soft, about 2–3 minutes.

2. Reduce heat to medium-low; add remaining ingredients except spinach. Stir well to combine.

3. Simmer on low heat, uncovered, stirring occasionally, for 8–10 minutes.

4. Add spinach and allow to cook for another 1–2 minutes, just until spinach is wilted.

5. Remove from heat and adjust seasonings to taste. Soup will thicken as it cools.

PER SERVING Calories: 408 | Fat: 24g | Sodium: 1,202mg | Fiber: 8g | Protein: 13g

Barley Vegetable Soup

Barley Vegetable Soup is an excellent "kitchen sink" recipe, meaning that you can toss in just about any fresh or frozen vegetables or spices you happen to have on hand.

INGREDIENTS | SERVES 6

1 onion, chopped
2 carrots, sliced
2 ribs celery, chopped
2 tablespoons olive oil
8 cups vegetable broth
1 cup barley, uncooked
1½ cups frozen mixed vegetables
1 (14-ounce) can crushed or diced tomatoes
½ teaspoon parsley
½ teaspoon thyme
2 bay leaves
Salt and pepper, to taste

1. In a large soup or stockpot, sauté the onion, carrots, and celery in olive oil for 3–5 minutes, just until onions are almost soft.

2. Reduce heat to medium low; add remaining ingredients except salt and pepper.

3. Bring to a simmer; cover, and allow to cook for at least 45 minutes, stirring occasionally.

4. Remove cover; allow to cook for 10 more minutes.

5. Remove bay leaves; season with salt and pepper to taste.

PER SERVING Calories: 228 | Fat: 5g | Sodium: 1,380mg | Fiber: 9g | Protein: 6g

Cream of Carrot Soup with Coconut

This carrot soup will knock your socks off! The addition of coconut milk transforms an ordinary carrot and ginger soup into an unexpected treat.

INGREDIENTS | SERVES 6

3 medium carrots, chopped
1 sweet potato, chopped
1 yellow onion, chopped
3½ cups vegetable broth
3 cloves garlic, minced
2 teaspoons fresh ginger, minced
1 (14-ounce) can coconut milk
1 teaspoon salt, or to taste
¾ teaspoon cinnamon (optional)

1. In a large soup or stockpot, bring the carrots, sweet potato, and onion to a simmer in the broth.

2. Add garlic and ginger; cover, and heat for 20–25 minutes, until carrots and potatoes are soft.

3. Allow to cool slightly; transfer to a blender, and purée until smooth.

4. Return soup to pot. Over very low heat, stir in the coconut milk and salt, stirring well to combine. Heat just until heated through, another 3–4 minutes.

5. Garnish with cinnamon just before serving.

PER SERVING Calories: 177 | Fat: 14g | Sodium: 978mg | Fiber: 2g | Protein: 2g

Easy Roasted Tomato Soup

Use the freshest, ripest, juiciest red tomatoes you can find for this super-easy recipe, as there are fewer other added flavors. If you find that you need a bit more spice, add a spoonful of nutritional yeast, a dash of cayenne pepper, or an extra shake of salt and pepper.

INGREDIENTS | SERVES 4

6 large tomatoes
1 small onion
4 cloves garlic
2 tablespoons olive oil
1¼ cups unflavored soymilk
2 tablespoons chopped fresh basil
1½ teaspoons balsamic vinegar
¾ teaspoon salt, or to taste
¼ teaspoon black pepper

1. Preheat oven to 425°F.

2. Slice tomatoes in half and chop onion into quarters. Place tomatoes, onion, and garlic on baking sheet and drizzle with olive oil.

3. Roast in the oven for 45 minutes to 1 hour.

4. Carefully transfer tomatoes, onion, and garlic to a blender, including any juices on the baking sheet. Add remaining ingredients; purée until almost smooth.

5. Reheat over low heat for 1–2 minutes if needed; adjust seasonings to taste.

PER SERVING Calories: 153 | Fat: 9g | Sodium: 488mg | Fiber: 4g | Protein: 5g

Indian Curried Lentil Soup

Similar to a traditional Indian lentil dal recipe, but with added vegetables to make it into an entrée, this lentil soup is perfect as is or paired with rice or some warmed Indian flatbread.

INGREDIENTS | SERVES 4

1 onion, diced
1 carrot, sliced
3 whole cloves
2 tablespoons vegan margarine
1 teaspoon cumin
1 teaspoon turmeric
1 cup yellow or green lentils, uncooked
2¾ cups vegetable broth
2 large tomatoes, chopped
1 teaspoon salt, or to taste
¼ teaspoon black pepper
1 teaspoon lemon juice

1. In a large soup or stockpot, sauté the onion, carrot, and cloves in margarine until onions are just turning soft, about 3 minutes. Add cumin and turmeric; toast for 1 minute, stirring constantly to avoid burning.

2. Reduce heat to medium-low; add lentils, broth, tomatoes, and salt. Bring to a simmer; cover, and cook for 35–40 minutes, or until lentils are done.

3. Season with black pepper and lemon juice just before serving.

PER SERVING Calories: 265 | Fat: 6g | Sodium: 1,328mg | Fiber: 17g | Protein: 14g

White Bean and Orzo Minestrone

Italian minestrone is a simple and universally loved soup.
This version uses tiny orzo pasta, cannellini beans, and plenty of veggies.

INGREDIENTS | SERVES 6

3 cloves garlic, minced

1 onion, chopped

2 ribs celery, chopped

2 tablespoons olive oil

5 cups vegetable broth

1 carrot, diced

1 cup green beans, chopped

2 small potatoes, chopped small

2 tomatoes, chopped

1 (15-ounce) can cannellini beans, drained and rinsed

1 teaspoon basil

½ teaspoon oregano

¾ cup orzo

Salt and pepper, to taste

1. In a large soup pot, heat garlic, onion, and celery in olive oil until just soft, about 3–4 minutes.

2. Add broth, carrot, green beans, potatoes, tomatoes, beans, basil, and oregano; bring to a simmer. Cover, and cook on medium-low heat for 20–25 minutes.

3. Add orzo; heat another 10 minutes, just until orzo is cooked. Season well with salt and pepper.

PER SERVING Calories: 304 | Fat: 5g | Sodium: 814mg | Fiber: 8g | Protein: 11g

Ten-Minute Cheater's Chili

No time? No problem! This is a quick and easy way to get some veggies and protein on the table with no hassle. Instead of veggie burgers, you could toss in a handful of TVP flakes, if you'd like, or any other mock meat you happen to have on hand.

INGREDIENTS | SERVES 4

1 (12-ounce) jar salsa

1 (14-ounce) can diced tomatoes

2 (14-ounce) cans kidney beans or black beans, drained and rinsed

1½ cups frozen mixed veggies

4 veggie burgers, crumbled (optional)

2 tablespoons chili powder

1 teaspoon cumin

½ cup water

1. In a large pot, combine all ingredients.

2. Simmer for 10 minutes, stirring frequently.

PER SERVING Calories: 271 | Fat: 3g | Sodium: 1,154mg | Fiber: 17g | Protein: 15g

Thai Tom Kha Coconut Soup

*In Thailand, this soup is a full meal, served alongside a large plate of steamed rice.
Don't worry if you can't find lemongrass or galangal, as lime and ginger add a similar flavor.*

INGREDIENTS | SERVES 4

1 (14-ounce) can coconut milk

2 cups vegetable broth

1 tablespoon soy sauce

3 cloves garlic, minced

5 slices fresh ginger or galangal

1 stalk lemongrass, chopped (optional)

1 tablespoon lime juice

1–2 small chilies, chopped

½ teaspoon red pepper flakes, or to taste

1 onion, chopped

2 tomatoes, chopped

1 carrot, sliced thin

½ cup sliced mushrooms, any kind

¼ cup chopped fresh cilantro

1. Over medium-low heat, combine the coconut milk and vegetable broth. Add soy sauce, garlic, ginger, lemongrass, lime juice, chilies, and red pepper flakes; heat for about 10 minutes, but do not boil.

2. When broth is hot, add onion, tomatoes, carrot, and mushrooms. Cover, and cook on low heat for 10–15 minutes.

3. Remove from heat; top with chopped fresh cilantro.

PER SERVING Calories: 240 | Fat: 21g | Sodium: 725mg | Fiber: 2g | Protein: 4g

Cold Spanish Gazpacho with Avocado

Best enjoyed on an outdoor patio just after sunset on a warm summer evening. But really, anytime you want a simple light starter soup will do, no matter the weather. Add some crunch by topping with homemade croutons.

INGREDIENTS | SERVES 6

2 cucumbers, diced

½ red onion, diced

2 large tomatoes, diced

¼ cup fresh chopped cilantro

2 avocados, diced

4 cloves garlic

2 tablespoons lime juice

1 tablespoon red wine vinegar

¾ cup vegetable broth

1 chili pepper (jalapeño, serrano, or cayenne) or 1 teaspoon hot sauce

Salt and pepper, to taste

1. Mix together the cucumbers, red onion, tomatoes, cilantro, and avocado. Set half of the mixture aside.

2. In a blender, mix the other half of the vegetable mixture. Add the garlic, lime juice, vinegar, vegetable broth, and chili pepper; process until smooth.

3. Transfer to serving bowl; add remaining diced cucumbers, onion, tomatoes, cilantro, and avocado, stirring gently to combine.

4. Season with salt and pepper, to taste.

PER SERVING Calories: 149 | Fat: 10g | Sodium: 130mg | Fiber: 7g | Protein: 3g

Kidney Bean and Zucchini Gumbo

This vegetable gumbo uses zucchini instead of okra. Traditional gumbo always calls for filé powder, but if you can't find this anywhere, increase the amounts of the other spices.

INGREDIENTS | SERVES 5

1 onion, diced
1 red or green bell pepper, chopped
3 stalks celery, chopped
2 tablespoons olive oil
1 zucchini, sliced
1 (14-ounce) can diced tomatoes
3 cups vegetable broth
1 teaspoon hot sauce
1 teaspoon filé powder (optional)
¾ teaspoon thyme
1 teaspoon Cajun seasoning
2 bay leaves
1 (15-ounce) can kidney beans, drained and rinsed
1½ cups cooked rice

1. In a large soup or stockpot, sauté the onion, bell pepper, and celery in olive oil for 1–2 minutes. Reduce heat; add remaining ingredients, except rice and beans.

2. Bring to a simmer; cover, and allow to cook for 30 minutes.

3. Uncover; add beans, and stir to combine. Heat for 5 more minutes.

4. Remove bay leaves before serving. Serve over cooked rice.

PER SERVING Calories: 227 | Fat: 6g | Sodium: 1,128mg | Fiber: 7g | Protein: 7g

Potato and Leek Soup

With simple earthy flavors, this classic soup is a comforting starter.

INGREDIENTS | SERVES 6

1 yellow onion, diced
2 cloves garlic, minced
2 tablespoons olive oil
6 cups vegetable broth
3 leeks, sliced
2 large potatoes, chopped
2 bay leaves
1 cup unflavored soymilk
2 tablespoons vegan margarine
¾ teaspoon salt, or to taste
⅓ teaspoon black pepper
½ teaspoon sage
½ teaspoon thyme
2 tablespoons nutritional yeast (optional)

1. Sauté onions and garlic in olive oil for 1–2 minutes, until onions are soft.

2. Add broth, leeks, potatoes, and bay leaves; bring to a slow simmer. Cook, partially covered, for 30 minutes, until potatoes are soft.

3. Remove bay leaves. Working in batches as needed, purée soup in a blender until almost smooth, or desired consistency.

4. Return soup to pot; stir in remaining ingredients. Adjust seasonings; reheat as needed.

PER SERVING Calories: 223 | Fat: 9g | Sodium: 1,321mg | Fiber: 4g | Protein: 4g

Cannellini Bean and Corn Chowder

This is a filling and textured soup that could easily be a main dish. Some chopped collards or a dash of hot sauce would be a welcome addition. For a lower fat version, skip the initial sauté and add about 5 minutes to the cooking time.

INGREDIENTS | SERVES 4

1 potato, chopped small

1 onion, chopped

2 tablespoons olive oil

3 cups vegetable broth

2 ears of corn, kernels cut off, or 1½ cups frozen or canned corn

1 (14-ounce) can cannellini or great northern beans, drained and rinsed

½ teaspoon thyme

¼ teaspoon black pepper

1 tablespoon flour

1½ cups unflavored soymilk

1. In a large soup or stockpot, sauté potato and onion in olive oil for 3–5 minutes.

2. Reduce heat and add vegetable broth. Bring to a slow simmer; cover, and allow to cook for 15–20 minutes.

3. Uncover; add corn, beans, thyme, and pepper.

4. Whisk together flour and soymilk; add to the pot, stirring well to prevent lumps.

5. Reduce heat to prevent soymilk from curdling; cook, uncovered, for 5–6 more minutes, stirring frequently.

6. Allow to cool slightly before serving, as soup will thicken as it cools.

PER SERVING Calories: 322 | Fat: 9g | Sodium: 761mg | Fiber: 8g | Protein: 13g

Super "Meaty" Chili with TVP

Any mock meat will work well in a vegetarian chili, but TVP is easy to keep on hand and very inexpensive. This is more of a thick, "meaty" Texas chili than a vegetable chili, but chili is easy and forgiving, so if you want to toss in some zucchini, broccoli, or diced carrots, by all means, do!

INGREDIENTS | SERVES 6

1½ cups TVP granules

1 cup hot vegetable broth

1 tablespoon soy sauce

1 yellow onion, chopped

5 cloves garlic, minced

2 tablespoons olive oil

1 cup corn kernels, fresh, frozen, or canned

1 bell pepper, any color, chopped

2 (15-ounce) cans black, kidney, or pinto beans, drained and rinsed

1 (15-ounce) can diced tomatoes

1 jalapeño pepper, minced, or ½ teaspoon cayenne pepper (optional)

1 teaspoon cumin

2 tablespoons chili powder

Salt and pepper, to taste

1. Cover the TVP with hot broth and soy sauce. Allow to sit for 3–4 minutes only, then drain.

2. In a large soup or stockpot, sauté the onion and garlic in olive oil until onions are soft, about 3–4 minutes.

3. Add remaining ingredients and TVP, stirring well to combine.

4. Cover, and allow to simmer over low heat for at least 30 minutes, stirring occasionally. Adjust seasonings to taste.

PER SERVING Calories: 272 | Fat: 6g | Sodium: 603mg | Fiber: 13g | Protein: 20g

Chinese Hot and Sour Soup

If you can't get enough of old Jackie Chan flicks and Wong Kar-wai films,
then this traditional Chinese soup is for you.

INGREDIENTS | SERVES 6

2 cups seitan, diced small, or other meat substitute

2 tablespoons vegetable oil

1½ teaspoons hot sauce

6 cups vegetable broth

½ head Napa cabbage, shredded

¾ cup sliced shiitake mushrooms

1 small can bamboo shoots, drained

2 tablespoons soy sauce

2 tablespoons white vinegar

¾ teaspoon crushed red pepper flakes

¾ teaspoon salt, or to taste

2 tablespoons cornstarch

¼ cup water

3 scallions, sliced

2 teaspoons sesame oil

1. Brown seitan in vegetable oil for 2–3 minutes, until cooked. Reduce heat to low; add hot sauce, stirring well to coat. Cook over low heat for 1 more minute; remove from heat and set aside.

2. In a large soup or stockpot, combine broth, cabbage, mushrooms, bamboo, soy sauce, vinegar, red pepper, and salt. Bring to a slow simmer and cover. Simmer for at least 15 minutes.

3. In a separate small bowl, whisk together the cornstarch and water; slowly stir into soup. Heat just until soup thickens, about 3–5 minutes.

4. Portion into serving bowls; top each serving with scallions and drizzle with sesame oil.

PER SERVING Calories: 195 | Fat: 7g | Sodium: 1,927mg | Fiber: 3g | Protein: 18g

Curried Pumpkin Soup

You don't have to wait for fall to make this pumpkin soup, as canned pumpkin purée will work just fine. It's also excellent with coconut milk instead of soymilk.

INGREDIENTS | SERVES 4

1 yellow onion, diced

3 cloves garlic, minced

2 tablespoons vegan margarine

1 (15-ounce) can pumpkin purée

3 cups vegetable broth

2 bay leaves

1 tablespoon curry powder

1 teaspoon cumin

½ teaspoon ground ginger

1 cup unflavored soymilk

¼ teaspoon salt, or to taste

1. In a large soup or stockpot, heat onion and garlic in margarine until onion is soft, about 4–5 minutes.

2. Add pumpkin and broth; stir well to combine. Add bay leaves, curry, cumin, and ginger; bring to a slow simmer.

3. Cover and allow to cook for 15 minutes.

4. Reduce heat to low; add soymilk, stirring to combine. Heat for 1–2 minutes, or until heated through.

5. Season with salt, to taste; remove bay leaves before serving.

PER SERVING Calories: 136 | Fat: 7g | Sodium: 1,112mg | Fiber: 4g | Protein: 3g

Udon Noodle Buddha Bowl

This is a nutritious full meal in a bowl, which might be particularly comforting on the edge of a cold or after an early morning meditation. For an authentic Japanese flavor, add a large piece of kombu seaweed to the broth or use a vegetarian dashi stock (Chapter 21).

INGREDIENTS | SERVES 4

2 (8-ounce) packages udon noodles

3½ cups Shiitake and Garlic Broth (Chapter 21)

1½ teaspoons fresh minced ginger

1 tablespoon sugar

1 tablespoon soy sauce

1 tablespoon rice vinegar

¼ teaspoon red pepper flakes, or to taste

1 baby bok choy, sliced

1 cup mushrooms, any kind, sliced

1 (12-ounce) block silken tofu, cubed

¼ cup bean sprouts

1 cup fresh spinach

1 teaspoon sesame oil or hot chili oil

1. Cook noodles in boiling water until soft, about 5 minutes. Drain and divide into 4 serving bowls; set aside.

2. In a large pot, combine the Shiitake and Garlic Broth, ginger, sugar, soy sauce, vinegar, and red pepper flakes; bring to a simmer.

3. Add bok choy, mushrooms, and tofu; cook just until veggies are soft, about 10 minutes.

4. Add bean sprouts and spinach; simmer for 1 more minute, until spinach has wilted.

5. Remove from heat; drizzle with sesame oil or chili oil.

6. Divide soup into the 4 bowls containing cooked noodles; serve immediately.

PER SERVING Calories: 240 | Fat: 4g | Sodium: 453mg | Fiber: 1g | Protein: 12g

Winter Seitan Stew

If you're used to a "meat and potatoes" kind of diet, this hearty seitan and potato stew ought to become a favorite.

INGREDIENTS | SERVES 6

2 cups chopped seitan

1 onion, chopped

2 carrots, chopped

2 stalks celery, chopped

2 tablespoons olive oil

4 cups vegetable broth

2 potatoes, chopped

½ teaspoon sage

½ teaspoon rosemary

½ teaspoon thyme

2 tablespoons cornstarch

⅓ cup water

Salt and pepper, to taste

1. In a large soup pot, heat seitan, onion, carrots, and celery in olive oil for 4–5 minutes, stirring frequently, until seitan is lightly browned.

2. Add vegetable broth and potatoes; bring to a boil.

3. Reduce to a simmer; add spices, and cover. Allow to cook for 25–30 minutes, until potatoes are soft.

4. In a small bowl, whisk together cornstarch and water. Add to soup; stir to combine.

5. Cook, uncovered, for another 5–7 minutes, until stew has thickened.

6. Season with salt and pepper, to taste.

PER SERVING Calories: 213 | Fat: 6g | Sodium: 974mg | Fiber: 4g | Protein: 17g

CHAPTER 22

Snacks and Desserts

Strawberry Coconut Ice Cream

Rich and creamy, this is the most decadent dairy-free strawberry ice cream you'll ever taste.

INGREDIENTS | SERVES 6

2 cups coconut cream
1¾ cups frozen strawberries
¾ cup sugar
2 teaspoons vanilla
¼ teaspoon salt

1. Purée together all ingredients until smooth and creamy.

2. Transfer mixture to a large freezer-proof baking or casserole dish; freeze.

3. Stir every 30 minutes, until a smooth ice cream forms, about 4 hours. If mixture gets too firm, transfer to a blender, process until smooth, then return to freezer.

PER SERVING Calories: 475 | Fat: 16g | Sodium: 134mg | Fiber: 2g | Protein: 1g

Black Bean Guacamole

Sneaking some extra fiber and protein into a traditional Mexican guacamole makes this dip a more nutritious snack or appetizer.

INGREDIENTS | YIELDS 2 CUPS

1 (15-ounce) can black beans, drained and rinsed
3 avocados, pitted
1 tablespoon lime juice
3 scallions, chopped
1 large tomato, diced
2 cloves garlic, minced
½ teaspoon chili powder
¼ teaspoon salt, or to taste
1 tablespoon chopped fresh cilantro

1. In a medium-sized bowl, using a fork or a potato masher, mash the beans just until they are halfway mashed, leaving some texture.

2. Add the remaining ingredients; mash together until mixed.

3. Adjust seasonings to taste.

4. Allow to sit for at least 10 minutes before serving to allow the flavors to set.

5. Gently mix again just before serving.

PER ¼ CUP Calories: 198 | Fat: 11g | Sodium: 206mg | Fiber: 10g | Protein: 7g

Easy Vegan Pizza Bagels

Need a quick lunch or after-work snack? Pizza bagels to the rescue!
For a real treat, shop for vegetarian "pepperoni" slices to top it off!

INGREDIENTS | SERVES 4

⅓ cup vegan pizza sauce or tomato sauce

½ teaspoon garlic powder

¼ teaspoon salt, or to taste

½ teaspoon basil

½ teaspoon oregano

4 vegan bagels, sliced in half

8 slices vegan cheese or 1 cup grated vegan cheese

¼ cup sliced mushrooms (optional)

¼ cup sliced black olives

1. Preheat oven to 325°F.

2. Combine pizza sauce, garlic powder, salt, basil, and oregano.

3. Spread sauce over each bagel half; top with cheese, mushrooms, olives, or any other toppings.

4. Heat in oven for 8–10 minutes, or until cheese is melted.

PER SERVING Calories: 308 | Fat: 9g | Sodium: 900mg | Fiber: 2g | Protein: 13g

Eggplant Baba Ghanoush

Whip up a batch of Eggplant Baba Ghanoush, Roasted Red Pepper Hummus (Chapter 22), and some
Vegan Tzatziki (Chapter 22) and make a Mediterranean appetizer spread. Don't forget some vegan pita
bread to dip into your Baba.

INGREDIENTS | YIELDS 1½ CUPS

2 medium eggplants

3 tablespoons olive oil, divided

2 tablespoons lemon juice

¼ cup tahini

3 cloves garlic, minced

½ teaspoon cumin

½ teaspoon chili powder (optional)

¼ teaspoon salt, or to taste

1 tablespoon chopped fresh parsley

1. Preheat oven to 400°F.

2. Slice eggplants in half; prick several times with a fork.

3. Place on a baking sheet; drizzle with 1 tablespoon olive oil. Bake for 30 minutes, or until soft. Allow to cool slightly.

4. Remove inner flesh; place in a bowl.

5. Using a large fork or potato masher, mash eggplant together with remaining ingredients until almost smooth.

6. Adjust seasonings, to taste.

PER ¼ CUP Calories: 161 | Fat: 13g | Sodium: 113mg | Fiber: 6g | Protein: 3g

Green and Black Olive Tapenade

This olive tapenade can be used as a spread or dip for baguettes or crackers. If you don't have a food processor, you could also mash the ingredients together with a mortar and pestle or a large fork.

INGREDIENTS | YIELDS 1 CUP

½ cup green olives

¾ cup black olives

2 cloves garlic

1 tablespoon capers (optional)

2 tablespoons lemon juice

2 tablespoons olive oil

¼ teaspoon oregano

¼ teaspoon black pepper

Process all ingredients in a food processor until almost smooth.

PER TABLESPOON Calories: 29 | Fat: 3g | Sodium: 116mg | Fiber: 0g | Protein: 0g

Hot Artichoke Spinach Dip

Serve this creamy dip hot with some baguette slices, crackers, pita bread, or sliced bell peppers and jicama. If you want to get fancy, you can carve out a bread bowl for an edible serving dish.

INGREDIENTS | SERVES 8

1 (12-ounce) package frozen spinach, thawed

1 (14-ounce) can artichoke hearts, drained

¼ cup vegan margarine

¼ cup flour

2 cups soymilk

½ cup nutritional yeast

1 teaspoon garlic powder

1½ teaspoons onion powder

¼ teaspoon salt, or to taste

1. Preheat oven to 350°F. Purée spinach and artichokes together until almost smooth; set aside.

2. In a small saucepan, melt the margarine over low heat. Slowly whisk in flour, 1 tablespoon at a time, stirring constantly to avoid lumps, until thick, about 1–3 minutes.

3. Remove from heat and add spinach and artichoke mixture; stir to combine. Add remaining ingredients.

4. Transfer to an ovenproof casserole dish or bowl; bake for 20 minutes. Serve hot.

PER SERVING Calories: 134 | Fat: 7g | Sodium: 378mg | Fiber: 4g | Protein: 6g

Mango Citrus Salsa

Salsa has a variety of uses, and this recipe adds color and variety to your usual chips and dip or Mexican dishes.

INGREDIENTS | YIELDS 2 CUPS

1 mango, peeled and chopped
2 tangerines, peeled and chopped
½ red bell pepper, chopped
½ red onion, minced
3 cloves garlic, minced
½ jalapeño pepper, minced
2 tablespoons lime juice
½ teaspoon salt, or to taste
¼ teaspoon black pepper
3 tablespoons chopped fresh cilantro

1. Gently toss together all ingredients.

2. Allow to sit for at least 15 minutes before serving to allow flavors to mingle.

PER ¼ CUP Calories: 37 | Fat: 0g | Sodium: 147mg | Fiber: 1g | Protein: 1g

Roasted Cashew and Spicy Basil Pesto

The combination of spicy purple Thai basil or holy basil instead of Italian sweet basil and the bite of the garlic creates an electrifying vegan pesto.

INGREDIENTS | SERVES 3

4 cloves garlic
1 cup Thai basil or holy basil, packed
⅔ cup roasted cashews
½ cup nutritional yeast
¾ teaspoon salt, or to taste
½ teaspoon black pepper
⅓–½ cup olive oil

1. In a blender or food processor, process all ingredients except olive oil just until coarse and combined.

2. Slowly incorporate olive oil until desired consistency is reached.

PER SERVING Calories: 435 | Fat: 38g | Sodium: 779mg | Fiber: 4g | Protein: 10g

Roasted Red Pepper Hummus

You'll rarely meet a vegan who doesn't love hummus in one form or another. As a veggie dip or sandwich spread, hummus is always a favorite. Up the garlic in this recipe, if that's your thing, and don't be ashamed to lick the spoons or spatula.

INGREDIENTS | YIELDS 1½ CUPS

1 (15-ounce) can chickpeas, drained and rinsed

⅓ cup tahini

⅔ cup chopped roasted red peppers

3 tablespoons lemon juice

2 tablespoons olive oil

2 cloves garlic

½ teaspoon cumin

⅓ teaspoon salt, or to taste

¼ teaspoon cayenne pepper (optional)

In a blender or food processor, process all ingredients until smooth, scraping the sides down as needed.

PER TABLESPOON Calories: 53 | Fat: 3g | Sodium: 110mg | Fiber: 1g | Protein: 1g

Tropical Cashew Nut Butter

You can make a homemade cashew nut butter with any kind of oil, so feel free to substitute using whatever you have on hand. But you're in for a real treat when you use coconut oil in this recipe!

INGREDIENTS | YIELDS ¾ CUP

2 cups roasted cashews

½ teaspoon sugar (optional)

¼ teaspoon salt (optional)

3–4 tablespoons coconut oil or other vegetable oil

1. In a food processor on high speed, process the cashews, sugar, and salt until finely ground. Continue processing until cashews form a thick paste.

2. Slowly add coconut oil until smooth and creamy, scraping down sides and adding a little more oil as needed.

PER 2 TABLESPOONS Calories: 320 | Fat: 28g | Sodium: 7mg | Fiber: 1g | Protein: 7g

Fresh Basil Bruschetta with Balsamic Reduction

Your guests will be so delighted by the rich flavors of the balsamic reduction sauce that they won't even notice that the cheese is missing from this vegan bruschetta. Use a fresh artisan bread, if you can, for extra flavor.

INGREDIENTS | SERVES 4

8–10 slices vegan French bread
¾ cup balsamic vinegar
1 tablespoon sugar
2 large tomatoes, diced small
3 cloves garlic, minced
2 tablespoons olive oil
¼ cup chopped fresh basil
Salt and pepper, to taste

1. Toast bread in toaster or for 5 minutes in the oven at 350°F.

2. In a small saucepan, whisk together the balsamic vinegar and sugar. Bring to a boil; reduce to a slow simmer. Allow to cook for 6–8 minutes, until almost thickened. Remove from heat.

3. In a large bowl, combine the tomatoes, garlic, olive oil, basil, salt, and pepper; gently toss with balsamic sauce.

4. Spoon tomato and balsamic mixture over bread slices; serve immediately.

PER SERVING Calories: 321 | Fat: 8g | Sodium: 434mg | Fiber: 3g | Protein: 9g

Mushroom Fondue

Nutritional yeast lends a rich flavor to this fun party fondue. If you don't have a fondue pot, you can mix the ingredients over low heat and serve hot. Don't forget plenty of dippers—vegan French bread, mushrooms, or lightly cooked baby potatoes would work well.

INGREDIENTS | SERVES 4

2 tablespoons vegan margarine
2 cups sliced mushrooms
½ cup unflavored soymilk or soy cream
1 teaspoon onion powder
½ teaspoon garlic powder
½ teaspoon celery salt
2 tablespoons flour
3 tablespoons nutritional yeast

1. Melt the margarine over low heat; add mushrooms. Allow to cook for 5 minutes, then add soymilk, onion powder, garlic powder, and celery salt. Cook for 8–10 minutes, until mushrooms are soft.

2. Allow mixture to cool slightly; purée in a blender.

3. Place puréed mushrooms in a fondue pot.

4. Over medium heat, whisk in flour; heat until thickened, about 2–4 minutes.

5. Stir in nutritional yeast; serve immediately.

PER SERVING Calories: 99 | Fat: 6g | Sodium: 163mg | Fiber: 1g | Protein: 4g

Vegan Cheese Ball

Use this recipe to make one impressive-looking large cheese ball, a cheese log, or make individual bite-sized servings for a party or the holidays. Everyone will be asking you for the recipe!

INGREDIENTS | MAKES 1 LARGE CHEESE BALL OR 12–14 BITE-SIZED CHEESE BALLS

1 block vegan nacho or Cheddar cheese, room temperature

1 container vegan cream cheese, room temperature

1 teaspoon garlic powder

½ teaspoon hot sauce

¼ teaspoon salt, or to taste

1 teaspoon paprika

¼ cup nuts, finely chopped

1. Grate cheese into a large bowl, or process in a food processor until finely minced. Using a large fork, mash the cheese together with the cream cheese, garlic powder, hot sauce, and salt until well mixed. (You may need to use your hands for this.)

2. Chill until firm, at least 1 hour; shape into ball or log shape, pressing firmly.

3. Sprinkle with paprika; carefully roll in nuts. Serve with crackers.

PER 1 BITE-SIZED CHEESE BALL Calories: 132 | Fat: 10g | Sodium: 285mg | Fiber: 2g | Protein: 2g

Vegan Chocolate Hazelnut Spread

Treat yourself or your family with this rich, sticky chocolate spread. This one will have you dancing around the kitchen and licking your spoons!

INGREDIENTS | YIELDS 1 CUP

2 cups hazelnuts, chopped

½ cup cocoa powder

¾ cup powdered sugar

½ teaspoon vanilla

4–5 tablespoons vegetable oil

1. In a food processor, process hazelnuts until very finely ground, about 3–4 minutes.

2. Add cocoa powder, sugar, and vanilla; process to combine.

3. Add oil, a little bit at a time, until mixture is soft and creamy and desired consistency is reached. You may need to add a bit more or less than 4–5 tablespoons.

PER TABLESPOON Calories: 164 | Fat: 14g | Sodium: 1mg | Fiber: 3g | Protein: 3g

Vegan Tzatziki

Use a vegan soy yogurt to make this classic Greek dip, which is best served very cold.
A nondairy sour cream may be used instead of the soy yogurt, if you prefer.

INGREDIENTS | YIELDS 1½ CUPS

1½ cups vegan soy yogurt, plain or lemon flavored
1 tablespoon olive oil
1 tablespoon lemon juice
4 cloves garlic, minced
2 cucumbers, grated or chopped fine
1 tablespoon chopped fresh mint or fresh dill

1. Whisk together yogurt, olive oil, and lemon juice until well combined.

2. Combine with remaining ingredients.

3. Chill for at least 1 hour before serving to allow flavors to mingle. Serve cold.

PER ¼ CUP Calories: 76 | Fat: 3g | Sodium: 10mg | Fiber: 1g | Protein: 2g

Apricot Ginger Sorbet

Made with real fruit and without dairy, this is a nearly fat-free treat that you
can add to smoothies or just enjoy outside on a hot summer day.

INGREDIENTS | SERVES 6

⅔ cup water
⅔ cup sugar
2 teaspoons fresh minced ginger
5 cups chopped apricots, fresh or frozen
3 tablespoons lemon juice

1. Bring the water, sugar, and ginger to a boil; reduce to a slow simmer. Heat for 3–4 more minutes, until sugar is dissolved and a syrup forms. Allow to cool.

2. Purée the sugar syrup, apricots, and lemon juice until smooth.

3. Transfer mixture to a large freezer-proof baking or casserole dish; freeze.

4. Stir every 30 minutes, until a smooth ice cream forms, about 4 hours. If mixture gets too firm, transfer to a blender, process until smooth, then return to freezer.

PER SERVING Calories: 154 | Fat: 1g | Sodium: 2mg | Fiber: 3g | Protein: 2g

Chocolate Peanut Butter Pudding

Whoever the genius was who first combined chocolate and peanut butter deserves a Nobel Prize. Or at least a MacArthur genius award.

INGREDIENTS | SERVES 4

1 (12-ounce) block silken tofu
¼ cup cocoa powder
½ teaspoon vanilla
¼ cup peanut butter or other nut butter
¼ cup maple syrup or brown rice syrup

Process all ingredients together until smooth and creamy.

PER SERVING Calories: 195 | Fat: 10g | Sodium: 80mg | Fiber: 1g | Protein: 8g

Coconut Rice Pudding

The combination of juicy soft mango with tropical coconut milk is simply heavenly, but if mangos are unavailable, pineapples or strawberries would add a delicious touch to this refined lightly sweetened dessert.

INGREDIENTS | SERVES 4

1½ cups cooked white rice
1½ cups vanilla soymilk
1½ cups coconut milk
3 tablespoons brown rice syrup or maple syrup
2 tablespoons agave nectar
4–5 dates, chopped
Dash cinnamon or nutmeg
2 mangos, chopped

1. Combine rice, soymilk, and coconut milk over low heat. Bring to a very low simmer for 10 minutes, or until mixture starts to thicken.

2. Stir in brown rice syrup, agave nectar, and dates; heat for another 2–3 minutes.

3. Allow to cool slightly before serving to allow pudding to thicken slightly. Garnish with a dash of cinnamon and fresh fruit just before serving.

PER SERVING Calories: 448 | Fat: 20g | Sodium: 51mg | Fiber: 3g | Protein: 6g

Easy Banana Date Cookies

The daily fast during Ramadan is traditionally broken with a date at sunset, and a version of these simple, refined sugar–free cookies is popular in Islamic communities in northern Africa, though almonds are traditionally added.

INGREDIENTS | YIELDS 1 DOZEN COOKIES

1 cup chopped pitted dates
1 banana, medium ripe
¼ teaspoon vanilla
1¾ cups coconut flakes

1. Preheat oven to 375°F. Cover dates in water and soak for about 10 minutes, until softened. Drain.

2. Process the dates, banana, and vanilla until almost smooth. Stir in coconut flakes by hand until thick. You may need a little more or less than 1¾ cups.

3. Drop by generous tablespoonfuls onto a cookie sheet. Bake 10–12 minutes, or until done. Cookies will be soft and chewy.

PER 1 COOKIE Calories: 111 | Fat: 6g | Sodium: 4mg | Fiber: 3g | Protein: 1g

Chocolate Mocha Ice Cream

If you have an ice-cream maker, you can skip the stirring and freezing and just add the blended ingredients to your machine.

INGREDIENTS | SERVES 6

1 cup vegan chocolate chips
1 cup soymilk
1 (12-ounce) block silken tofu
⅓ cup sugar
2 tablespoons instant coffee
2 teaspoons vanilla
¼ teaspoon salt

1. Using a double broiler, or over very low heat, melt chocolate chips until smooth and creamy, about 5 minutes. Allow to cool slightly.

2. Blend together the soymilk, tofu, sugar, coffee, vanilla, and salt until smooth, at least 2 minutes.

3. Add melted chocolate chips; process until smooth.

4. Transfer mixture to a large freezer-proof baking or casserole dish; freeze.

5. Stir every 30 minutes, until a smooth ice cream forms, about 4 hours. If mixture gets too firm, transfer to a blender, process until smooth, then return to freezer.

PER SERVING Calories: 150 | Fat: 8g | Sodium: 120mg | Fiber: 0g | Protein: 5g

No-Bake Cocoa Balls

Craving a healthy chocolate snack? Try these fudgy little cocoa balls,
similar to a soft no-bake cookie, but with no refined sugar.

INGREDIENTS | SERVES 4

1 cup chopped pitted dates
1 cup walnuts or cashews
¼ cup cocoa powder
1 tablespoon peanut butter
¼ cup coconut flakes

Variations

Roll these little balls in extra coconut flakes for a sweet presentation, or try it with carob powder instead of cocoa—they're just as satisfying. Don't have fresh dates on hand? Raisins may be substituted, but skip the soaking. Even with raisins, you really won't believe they're sugar free.

1. Cover dates in water; soak for about 10 minutes, until softened. Drain.

2. In a food processor, process dates, nuts, cocoa powder, and peanut butter until combined and sticky.

3. Add coconut flakes; process until coarse.

4. Shape into balls; chill.

5. If mixture is too wet, add more nuts and coconut; add just a touch of water if the mixture is dry and crumbly.

PER SERVING Calories: 348 | Fat: 22g | Sodium: 23mg | Fiber: 8g | Protein: 7g

Chewy Oatmeal Raisin Cookies

The addition of applesauce keeps these classic nostalgic cookies super chewy.
No egg replacer needed.

INGREDIENTS | YIELDS 1½ DOZEN COOKIES

⅓ cup vegan margarine, softened
½ cup brown sugar
¼ cup sugar
⅓ cup applesauce
1 teaspoon vanilla
2 tablespoons soymilk
¾ cup whole-wheat flour
½ teaspoon baking soda
½ teaspoon cinnamon
½ teaspoon ginger
1¾ cups quick-cooking oats
⅔ cup raisins

1. Preheat oven to 350°F.

2. Beat the margarine and sugars together until smooth and creamy. Add applesauce, vanilla, and soymilk.

3. Sift together the flour, baking soda, cinnamon, and ginger; add to wet ingredients.

4. Stir in oats, then raisins; drop by generous spoonfuls onto a cookie sheet.

5. Bake for 10–12 minutes, or until done.

PER 1 COOKIE Calories: 122 | Fat: 4g | Sodium: 85mg | Fiber: 2g | Protein: 2g

Quinoa "Tapioca" Pudding

Instead of tapioca pudding or baked rice pudding, try this whole-grain version made with quinoa. Healthy enough to eat for breakfast, but sweet enough for dessert, too.

INGREDIENTS | SERVES 4

1 cup quinoa

2 cups water

2 cups soymilk or soy cream

2 tablespoons maple syrup or brown rice syrup

1 teaspoon cornstarch

2 bananas, sliced thin

½ teaspoon vanilla

⅓ cup raisins

Dash cinnamon or nutmeg (optional)

1. In a medium saucepan over medium heat, simmer quinoa in water, covered, stirring frequently, for 10–15 minutes, until done and water is absorbed.

2. Reduce heat to medium-low. Stir in soymilk, maple syrup, cornstarch, and bananas; combine well.

3. Heat, stirring constantly, for 6–8 minutes, until bananas are soft and pudding has thickened.

4. Stir in vanilla and raisins while still hot; sprinkle with a dash of cinnamon, to taste.

PER SERVING Calories: 325 | Fat: 5g | Sodium: 67mg | Fiber: 5g | Protein: 11g

Pumpkin Maple Pie

For Thanksgiving or any time, this pie supplies plenty of vitamin A from the pumpkin.

INGREDIENTS | SERVES 8

1 (16-ounce) can pumpkin purée

½ cup maple syrup

1 (12-ounce) block silken tofu

¼ cup sugar

1½ teaspoons cinnamon

½ teaspoon ginger powder

½ teaspoon nutmeg

¼ teaspoon ground cloves (optional)

½ teaspoon salt

1 vegan prepared pie crust

1. Preheat oven to 400°F.

2. Process the pumpkin, maple syrup, and tofu until smooth and creamy.

3. Add sugar and spices; pour into pie crust.

4. Bake for 1 hour, or until done. Allow to cool before slicing and serving, as pie will set and firm as it cools.

PER SERVING Calories: 266 | Fat: 9g | Sodium: 381mg | Fiber: 2g | Protein: 3g

Nacho "Cheese" Dip

Peanut butter in cheese sauce? No, that's not a typo! Just a touch of peanut butter creates a creamy and nutty layer of flavor to this sauce, and helps it to thicken nicely. Use this sauce to dress plain steamed veggies or make homemade nachos.

INGREDIENTS | YIELDS ABOUT 1 CUP

3 tablespoons vegan margarine
1 cup unsweetened soymilk
¾ teaspoon garlic powder
½ teaspoon salt, or to taste
½ teaspoon onion powder
1 tablespoon peanut butter
¼ cup flour
¼ cup nutritional yeast
¾ cup salsa
2 tablespoons chopped canned jalapeño peppers (optional)

1. In a pan over low heat, heat margarine and soymilk.

2. Add garlic powder, salt, and onion powder; stir to combine.

3. Add peanut butter; stir until melted.

4. Whisk in flour, 1 tablespoon at a time, until smooth. Heat until thickened, about 5–6 minutes.

5. Stir in nutritional yeast, salsa, and jalapeño peppers.

6. Allow to cool slightly before serving, as cheese sauce will thicken as it cools.

PER ¼ CUP Calories: 184 | Fat: 12g | Sodium: 725mg | Fiber: 3g | Protein: 6g

Classic Chocolate Chip Cookies

Just like mom used to make, only with a little applesauce to cut down on the fat a bit.

INGREDIENTS | YIELDS ABOUT 2 DOZEN COOKIES

⅔ cup vegan margarine
⅔ cup sugar
⅔ cup brown sugar
⅓ cup applesauce
1½ teaspoons vanilla
Egg replacer for 2 eggs
2½ cups flour
1 teaspoon baking soda
½ teaspoon baking powder
1 teaspoon salt
⅔ cup quick-cooking oats
1½ cups vegan chocolate chips

1. Preheat oven to 375°F.

2. In a large mixing bowl, cream together the margarine and white sugar; mix in brown sugar, applesauce, vanilla, and egg replacer.

3. In a separate bowl, combine the flour, baking soda, baking powder, and salt; combine with the wet ingredients. Mix well.

4. Stir in oats and chocolate chips just until combined.

5. Drop by generous spoonfuls onto a baking sheet; bake for 10–12 minutes.

PER 1 COOKIE Calories: 161 | Fat: 7g | Sodium: 232mg | Fiber: 1g | Protein: 2g

Avocado and Shiitake Pot Stickers

Once you try these California-fusion pot stickers, you'll wish you had made a double batch! These little dumplings don't need to be enhanced with a complex dipping sauce, so serve them plain or with soy sauce.

INGREDIENTS | YIELDS 12–15 POT STICKERS

1 avocado, diced small
½ cup shiitake mushrooms, diced
½ block (6 ounces) silken tofu, crumbled
1 clove garlic, minced
2 teaspoons balsamic vinegar
1 teaspoon soy sauce
12–15 vegan dumpling wrappers
Water for steaming or oil for pan frying

Whether Steamed or Fried . . .

In dumpling houses across East Asia, dumplings are served with a little bowl of freshly grated ginger, and diners create a simple dipping sauce from the various condiments on the table. To try it, pour some rice vinegar and a touch of soy sauce over a bit of ginger and add hot chili oil to taste.

1. In a small bowl, gently mash together all ingredients except wrappers, just until mixed and crumbly.

2. Place about 1½ teaspoons of the filling in the middle of each wrapper. Fold in half and pinch closed, forming little pleats. You may want to dip your fingertips in water to help the dumplings stay sealed, if needed.

3. To pan fry: Heat a thin layer of oil in a large skillet. Carefully add dumplings and cook for just 1 minute. Add about ½ cup water; cover, and cook for 3–4 minutes.

4. To steam: Carefully place a layer of dumplings in a steamer, being sure the dumplings don't touch. Place steamer above boiling water; allow to cook, covered, for 3–4 minutes.

PER 2 POT STICKERS (STEAMED) Calories: 304 | Fat: 6g | Sodium: 356mg | Fiber: 4g | Protein: 9g

Maple Date Carrot Cake

With applesauce for moisture and just a touch of oil, this is a cake you can feel good about eating for breakfast. Leave out the dates if you want even less natural sugar.

INGREDIENTS | SERVES 8

1½ cups raisins

1⅓ cups pineapple juice

6 dates, diced

2¼ cups grated carrot

½ cup maple syrup

¼ cup applesauce

2 tablespoons oil

3 cups flour

1½ teaspoons baking soda

½ teaspoon salt

1 teaspoon cinnamon

½ teaspoon allspice or nutmeg

Egg replacer for 2 eggs

1. Preheat oven to 375°F; grease and flour a cake pan.

2. Combine the raisins with pineapple juice; allow to sit for 5–10 minutes to soften.

3. In a separate small bowl, cover the dates with water until soft, about 10 minutes. Drain water.

4. In a large mixing bowl, combine the raisins and pineapple juice, carrot, maple syrup, applesauce, oil, and dates.

5. In a separate large bowl, combine the flour, baking soda, salt, cinnamon, and allspice.

6. Combine the dry ingredients with the wet ingredients; add prepared egg replacer. Mix well.

7. Pour batter into prepared cake pan; bake for 30 minutes, or until a toothpick inserted in the center comes out clean.

PER SERVING Calories: 394 | Fat: 4g | Sodium: 406mg | Fiber: 4g | Protein: 6g

Sweetheart Raspberry Lemon Cupcakes

Add ½ teaspoon of lemon extract for extra lemony goodness in these sweet and tart cupcakes. Or omit the raspberries and add 3 tablespoons of poppy seeds for lemon poppy seed cupcakes. Sweet and tart sweetheart! Get it?

INGREDIENTS | YIELDS 18 CUPCAKES

½ cup vegan margarine, softened
1 cup sugar
½ teaspoon vanilla
⅔ cup soymilk
3 tablespoons lemon juice
Zest from 2 lemons
1¾ cups flour
1½ teaspoons baking powder
½ teaspoon baking soda
¼ teaspoon salt
¾ cup diced raspberries, fresh or frozen

Raspberry Cream Cheese Frosting

Combine a half container of vegan cream cheese with ½ cup raspberry jam and 6 tablespoons of softened vegan margarine. Beat until smooth, then add powdered sugar until a creamy frosting forms. You'll need about 2½ cups. Pile it high and garnish your cupcakes with fresh strawberry slices or pink vegan candies.

1. Preheat oven to 350°F; grease or line a cupcake tin.

2. Beat together the margarine and sugar until light and fluffy.

3. Add vanilla, soymilk, lemon juice, and zest.

4. In a separate bowl, sift together the flour, baking powder, baking soda, and salt.

5. Combine flour mixture with wet ingredients just until mixed; do not overmix.

6. Gently fold in diced raspberries.

7. Fill cupcakes about ⅔ full with batter; bake immediately for 16–18 minutes, or until done.

PER 1 CUPCAKE Calories: 139 | Fat: 5g | Sodium: 182mg | Fiber: 1g | Protein: 2g

Additional Resources

ABCs of Pregnancy—General Pregnancy Information

Reliable, comprehensive sources of pregnancy information and support.

About Pregnancy and Childbirth
With Robin Elise Weiss, ICCE-CPE, CD (DONA)
http://pregnancy.about.com

Ask Dr. Sears
With Dr. Bill Sears and Martha Sears, RN
www.askdrsears.com

March of Dimes
Pregnancy and Newborn Health Education Center
www.marchofdimes.com

The Visible Embryo
A pictorial tour of embryonic and fetal development created with a grant from the National Institutes of Health (NIH).
www.visembryo.com

Childbirth Education

Find a childbirth educator or obtain more information on popular methods of childbirth. (See also "Professional Organizations")

HypnoBirthing
P.O. Box 810
Epsom, NH 03234
www.hypnobirthing.com

Lamaze International
2025 M Street, NW
Suite 800
Washington, DC 20036-3309
800-368-4404
www.lamaze.org

Marvelous Multiples
www.marvelousmultiples.com

Waterbirth International
P.O. Box 5578
Lighthouse Point, FL 33074
954-821-9125
www.waterbirth.org

Complications in Pregnancy

Educational resources and support for complications in pregnancy.

American Diabetes Association
More information on the diagnosis and treatment of gestational diabetes.
1-800-DIABETES (1-800-342-2383)
www.diabetes.org/diabetes-basics/gestational

Preeclampsia Foundation
6767 N Wickham Road, Suite 400
Melbourne, FL 32940
800-665-9341
www.preeclampsia.org

**Sidelines High Risk Pregnancy Support
National Office**
P.O. Box 1808
Laguna Beach, CA 92652
888-447-4754 (HI-RISK4)
www.sidelines.org

Having a Healthy Pregnancy

Resources for prenatal health.

Motherisk
The Hospital for Sick Children
555 University Avenue
Toronto, Ontario, Canada M5G 1X8
Alcohol and Substance Use Helpline:
877-327-4636
Nausea and Vomiting of Pregnancy Helpline:
800-436-8477
Motherisk Home Line: 416-813-6780
www.motherisk.org

The National Toxicology Program (NTP)
Center for the Evaluation of Risks to Human
Reproduction (CERHR)
NIEHS EC-32
P.O. Box 12233, MD K2-04
Research Triangle Park, NC 27709
919-541-5021
http://cerhr.niehs.nih.gov

Infant Health and Development

Essentials for a healthy start in life.

Keep Kids Healthy
A Pediatrician's Guide to Your Children's Health
and Safety
www.keepkidshealthy.com

KidsHealth
A Project of The Nemours Foundation
www.kidshealth.org

Zero to Three
National Center for Infants, Toddlers and Families
1255 23rd Street, NW, Suite 350
Washington, DC 20037
202-638-1144
www.zerotothree.org

Maternal and Infant Nutrition and Food Safety

Breastfeeding facts, support, and nutrition assistance before and after pregnancy.

Food Safety for Moms-To-Be
*www.fda.gov/food/resourcesforyou/
healtheducators/ucm081785.htm*

**International Lactation Consultant
Association**
2501 Aerial Center Parkway, Suite 103
Morrisville, NC 27560
1-888-ILCA-IS-U
www.ilca.org

La Leche League International
957 N. Plum Grove Road
Schaumburg, IL 60173
1-800-LALECHE
www.llli.org

ChooseMyPlate.gov
www.choosemyplate.gov

Women, Infants, and Children (WIC)
Supplemental Food Programs Division
Food and Nutrition Service
United States Department of Agriculture
3101 Park Center Drive
Alexandria, VA 22302
703-305-2746
www.fns.usda.gov/wic

Postpartum Health Issues

Learn more about common maternal health
issues occurring after birth.

American Thyroid Association
www.thyroid.org

Postpartum Support International
6706 SW 54th Ave.
Portland, OR 97219
800-944-4773 (800-944-4PPD)
www.postpartum.net

Professional Organizations

Need a referral? These professional organizations can help. (See also "Maternal and Infant
Nutrition")

**American Congress of Obstetricians and
Gynecologists (ACOG)**
Resource Center
P.O. Box 96920
Washington, DC 20090-6920
202-638-5577
www.acog.org

American College of Nurse-Midwives
8403 Colesville Road, Suite 1550
Silver Spring, MD 20910
240-485-1800
www.midwife.org

American Dietetic Association (ADA)
Find an RD
800-877-1600
www.eatright.org

Doulas of North America (DONA)
1582 S. Parker Rd., Suite 201
Denver, CO 80231
888-788-DONA (3662)
www.dona.org

**International Childbirth Education
Association (ICEA)**
1500 Sunday Drive, Suite 102
Raleigh, NC 27607
800-624-4934
www.icea.org

American Association of Birth Centers (AABC)
3123 Gottschall Road
Perkiomenville, PA 18074
866-54-BIRTH
www.birthcenters.org

National Society of Genetic Counselors (NSGC)
401 N. Michigan Ave., 22nd Floor
Chicago, IL 60611
312-321-6834
www.nsgc.org

Special Issues

Special issues in pregnancy and beyond.

Centers for Disease Control and Prevention—Emergency Preparedness and Response
Disaster Planning Resources
www.bt.cdc.gov

Hygeia Foundation, Inc.
An Institute for Perinatal Loss and Bereavement
264 Amity Rd., Suite 211
Woodbridge, CT 06525
1-800-893-9198
www.hygeiafoundation.org

International Cesarean Awareness Network (ICAN)
P.O. Box 98
Savage, MN 55378
1-800-686-ICAN
www.ican-online.org

National Down Syndrome Society (NDSS)
666 Broadway, 8th Floor
New York, NY 10012
800-221-4602
www.ndss.org

National Organization on Fetal Alcohol Syndrome (NOFAS)
1200 Eton Ct, NW, 3rd Floor
Washington, DC 20007
800-66NOFAS
www.nofas.org

Spina Bifida Association of America (SBAA)
4590 MacArthur Blvd., NW
Suite 250
Washington, DC 20007-4226
800-621-3141
www.spinabifidaassociation.org

Women's Health Information Center
Includes resources on pregnancy, birth options, and women's health issues.
www.womenshealth.gov

Twins or More

Resources for moms and dads of multiples. (See also "Childbirth Education")

About Parenting Multiples
With Pamela Prindle Fierro
http://multiples.about.com

Mothers of Supertwins (MOST)
P.O. Box 306
East Islip, NY 11730-0306
631-859-1110
www.mostonline.org

National Organization of Mothers of Twins Clubs Inc. (NOMOTC)
Executive Office
2000 Mallory Ln., Suite 130-600
Franklin, TN 37067-8231
248-231-4480
www.nomotc.org

Support for Single Mothers

Information and emotional support for unmarried mothers and moms-to-be.

National Organization of Single Mothers
www.singlemothers.org

Vegans

Resources especially for vegans.

American Dietetic Association's Position Paper: Vegetarian Diets
www.eatright.org/About/Content aspx?id=8357

Happy Cow: Vegetarian Restaurants Guide
www.happycow.net

Pangea Vegan Products
www.veganstore.com

North American Vegetarian Society (NAVS)
www.navs-online.org

Vegan Essentials—Online Vegan Store
www.veganessentials.com

Vegetarian Journal's Guide to Food Ingredients
www.vrg.org/ingredients/index.php

Vegetarian Nutrition Dietetic Practice Group
Consumer-friendly information from RDs with an interest in vegetarian nutrition.
www.vegetariannutrition.net

The Vegetarian Resource Group (VRG)
Nonprofit organization providing information about vegan living.
P.O. Box 1463
Baltimore, MD 21203
410-366-8343
www.vrg.org

Birth Plan Checklist

Consider starting your birth plan with a short note both to your provider and to the nursing staff that will be caring for you during labor and delivery. Explain your general wishes for a healthy and safe delivery, for joint decision making should medical interventions be required, and for open communication throughout the process. Read Chapter 14 to learn more about birth plans. Then use this checklist as a guide to assembling the basics.

1. Where will the birth take place?
1. Hospital
2. Birthing center
3. Home
4. Other:

2. Who will be there for labor support?
1. Husband or significant other
2. Doula
3. Friend
4. Family member

3. Will any room modifications or equipment be required to increase your comfort mentally and physically?
1. Objects from home (for example, pictures, blanket, pillow)
2. Lighting adjustments
3. Music
4. Video or photos of birth
5. Other:

4. Any special requests for labor prep procedures?
1. Forego enema
2. Self-administer the enema
3. Forego shaving
4. Shave self
5. Heparin lock instead of routine IV line
6. Other:

5. Eating and drinking during labor.
1. Want access to a light snack
2. Want access to water, sports drink, or other appropriate beverage
3. Want ice chips
4. Other:

6. Do you want pain medication?
1. Analgesic (for example, Stadol, Demerol, Nubain)
2. Epidural (If so, is timing an issue?)
3. Other:

7. What nonpharmaceutical pain-relief equipment might you want access to?
1. Hydrotherapy (shower, whirlpool)
2. Warm compresses
3. Birth ball
4. Other:

8. **What interventions would you like to avoid unless deemed a medical necessity by your provider during labor? Specify your preferred alternatives.**
   1. Episiotomy
   2. Forceps
   3. Internal fetal monitoring
   4. Pitocin (oxytocin)
   5. Other:

9. **What would you like your first face-to-face encounter with baby to be like?**
   1. Hold off on all nonessential treatment, evaluation, and tests for a specified time.
   2. If immediate tests and evaluation are necessary, you, your partner, or another support person will accompany baby.
   3. Want to nurse immediately following birth.
   4. Would like family members to meet baby immediately following birth.
   5. Other:

10. **If a cesarean birth is required, what is important to you and your partner?**
    1. Type of anesthesia (general versus spinal block)
    2. Having partner or another support person present
    3. Spending time with baby immediately following procedure
    4. Bonding with baby in the recovery room
    5. Type of postoperative pain relief and nursing considerations
    6. Other:

11. **Do you have a preference for who cuts the cord and when the cut is performed?**
    1. Mom
    2. Dad
    3. Provider
    4. Delay until cord stops pulsing
    5. Cord blood will be banked; cut per banking guidelines
    6. Cut at provider's discretion
    7. Other:

12. **What kind of postpartum care will you and baby have at the hospital?**
    1. Baby will room-in with mom.
    2. Baby will sleep in the nursery at night.
    3. Baby will breastfeed.
    4. Baby will bottle feed (indicate formula baby should be given).
    5. Baby will not be fed any supplemental formula and/or glucose water unless medically indicated.
    6. Baby will not be given a pacifier.
    7. Other:

13. **Considerations for after discharge**
    1. Support and short-term care for siblings
    2. Support if you've had a cesarean
    3. Maternity leave
    4. Other:

Index

RECIPES INDEX

Note: Page numbers in **bold** indicate recipe category lists.

We Have EVERYTHING® on Anything!

With more than 19 million copies sold, the Everything® series has become one of America's favorite resources for solving problems, learning new skills, and organizing lives. Our brand is not only recognizable—it's also welcomed.

The series is a hand-in-hand partner for people who are ready to tackle new subjects—like you!

For more information on the Everything® series, please visit *www.adamsmedia.com*

The Everything® list spans a wide range of subjects, with more than 500 titles covering 25 different categories:

Business	History	Reference
Careers	Home Improvement	Religion
Children's Storybooks	Everything Kids	Self-Help
Computers	Languages	Sports & Fitness
Cooking	Music	Travel
Crafts and Hobbies	New Age	Wedding
Education/Schools	Parenting	Writing
Games and Puzzles	Personal Finance	
Health	Pets	